The King and Queen are Naked

Establishment Failures
based on Scientific, Medical, and Psychiatric Research
on "Gender Dysphoria"

Stephen W. Rouhana, Ph.D.

En Route Books and Media, LLC
Saint Louis, MO

⊕*ENROUTE*
Make the time

En Route Books and Media, LLC

5705 Rhodes Avenue

St. Louis, MO 63109

Contact us at

contactus@enroutebooksandmedia.com

Cover Credit: Sebastian Mahfood using DALL-E

Copyright 2025 Stephen W. Rouhana

ISBN-13: 979-8-88870-453-0

Library of Congress Control Number:

Available online at https://catalog.loc.gov

DEDICATION

This book is dedicated to all those who struggle with gender dysphoria, and especially, for one *in pectore*. You may all rest assured of my daily prayers for your well-being.

LIST OF ABBREVIATIONS

AAP – American Academy of Pediatrics

ACE – Adverse Childhood Experience

AI – Asymmetry Index

AMA – American Medical Association

APA – American Psychiatric Association (NOT the American Psychological Association)

ASD – Autism Spectrum Disorder

BDD – Body Dysmorphic Disorder

BIID – Body Integrity Identity Disorder

CBCL – Child Behavior Checklist (can be Parent Report or YSR - Youth Self-Report)

CSH – Cross-Sex Hormones

DID – Dissociative Identity Disorder

DSM – Diagnostic and Statistical Manual of Mental Disorders

GICE – Gender Identity Conversion Efforts

GID – Gender Identity Disorder

GIDC – Gender Identity Disorder of Childhood

GD – "Gender Dysphoria"

GIV – Gender Identity Variation

HHS – refers to 2025 report on "Gender Dysphoria" by the US Health and Human Services Dept

ICD-XX – International Classification of Diseases (where XX refers to the revision number)

LGBT – Lesbian, Gay, Bisexual, and Transgender

MRI – Magnetic Resonance Imaging

PBs – Puberty Blockers

SOCE – Sexual Orientation Change Efforts
SRS – Sex "Reassignment" Surgery
WHO – World Health Organization
WPATH - World Professional Association for Transgender Health

ACKNOWLEDGMENTS

As for any work I have ever completed, this one has benefited tremendously from the help of others. Among others, I am especially thankful to the following individuals.

Dr. Mark Latkovic, may he rest in peace, moral theologian at Sacred Heart Major Seminary, who provided me with the first references on the issue of "Gender Dysphoria," and was kind enough to review and provide comments on the moral theology section in Part Three of this book in its earliest form.

Fr. Steven Mateja, Campus Minister for the Archdiocese of Detroit at Oakland University and Wayne State University, and a friend who provided me with early references on Church teaching about this subject.

A clinical psychologist from a university setting who reviewed the earliest manuscript and provided helpful comments but wishes to remain anonymous.

Dr. Monica Miller, who also reviewed and provided comments on an abridged form of the earliest manuscript.

Dr. Theresa Farnan, of the Ethics and Public Policy Center, who reviewed and provided comments on one of the later versions of the manuscript.

Fr. Peter Ryan, SJ, Professor of Theology, Fr. Michael J. McGivney Chair in Life Ethics at Sacred Heart Major Seminary, who provided comments on the moral theology aspects of the manuscript.

Mr. Robert Muise, Esq., who reviewed a more recent manuscript and provided critical comments that greatly improved the manuscript.

Dr. Paul Hruz, MD, PhD, Associate Professor of Pediatrics, Endocrinology & Diabetes and Associate Professor, Cell Biology & Physiology at Washington University School of Medicine, who reviewed the latest manuscript and who also provided critical comments that really helped improve the manuscript.

Dr. Duane DiFranco, Distinguished Fellow of the American Psychiatric Association, and former president of Michigan Psychiatric Society, who provided valuable input on the latest manuscript from a psychiatrist's perspective.

TABLE OF CONTENTS

PREFACE

At the beginning of the summer in 2015, we learned that a close young male friend of our family had decided that he was a female and was considering or had begun attempting to transition to the opposite sex with hormone treatments. He was one of my son's best friends during much of their childhood and came from a family of deep Catholic Faith and conviction. He himself was extremely well-formed in the Faith and was a brilliant young man who was still in love with the Lord. Our son was wondering what to do. He loved his friend and wanted to support him but was very conflicted.

I had no idea how to advise my son because I had only barely heard of such a thing and had no substantive knowledge on the subject. However, the previous December I had just retired from my 32-year long career, as a physicist, to discern a calling to the Diaconate and to finish a master's degree in Pastoral Studies. I had time on my hands and decided to learn as much as I could about this issue in hopes of being able to advise my son and in hopes of helping this young man and his family.

Immediately after we learned about this situation, I sent a moral theologian, from the Seminary at which I was studying, a request for any references or information he might have on this topic. He was kind enough to send me some links for journal articles and papers on the subject. After I received the references from him in June, with my background as a research scientist (PhD in Physics with a concentration in Biophysics), I started an aggressive literature search.

The more I read, the more apparent it was to me that there seemed to be no critical analysis of the "scholarly" papers in psychology that had been published, and that the APA (American Psychiatric Association) had lost its way. In addition, it was clear that there was no official, well-explained, Catholic position on the issue of "Gender Dysphoria," as the APA now refers to this condition. So, with my background as a research scientist, and as a master's level theologian, I delved into the scientific literature (Psychiatry, Psychology, and Medicine) and Church teachings. By the time I finished reading, I had read over 150 scientific papers and many magazine and other articles, I decided to write a paper pulling together all I had learned because I can process information better when I write about it. I tried to digest all the published work I could find and cite the most relevant literature in the paper. My hope was that it would clarify some of the issues and serve as a reference for people trying to understand this complex phenomenon.

So, over 5 months in 2015, I read over 150 technical reference papers and wrote a 40 page, single-spaced, size 10 font, review article to summarize what I had learned both from a scientific and faith standpoint. The article was titled "Toward Developing a Catholic View of Gender Dysphoria and Transgender Issues: Lessons from Scientific, Medical, and Psychiatric Research, Sacred Scripture, and the Catechism of the Catholic Church" (and yes, I know that sounds more like an abstract than a title).

It remains unpublished to this day for the following reason. While I believed my technical skills and religious training (Master of Arts in Pastoral Studies) had positioned me well to do this analysis, I also recognized that I am a physicist, not a psychologist or a psychiatrist. So, I started to send requests to people within the fields of psychology, psychiatry, and moral theology asking for a review. I didn't want to send it to a publisher without having some sort of review from those who are experts in the field.

The moral theologian who I had first contacted was kind enough to review that component of the manuscript for me and quickly provided me with comments. However, it took over two years to find a practicing clinical psychologist at a prominent research hospital who would review the article and provide comments to me. By the time I had that clinical psychologist review my article, it was too old to be submitted to a journal as a review article. I should note that the reviewer concluded that I had made no errors in my analysis dealing with the psychiatric or psychological matters.

At the beginning of summer in 2023, eight years later, given the social upheaval being wrought by this topic, I felt called, perhaps prompted by the Holy Spirit, to take up writing this article again. I considered it best to do another literature review to see if there were any major changes to the field. My new search was slightly more limited to approximately 125 new technical papers encompassing mostly scientific literature, in addition to some popular and/or religious articles. Interestingly, but not entirely unexpectedly, I found that much had remained the same. I decided to organize my original work into three parts. Part One covers the science of "Gender Dysphoria", insofar as there is any. The main focus of this part is whether or not the symptoms associated with "Gender Dysphoria" constitute a mental disorder. Part Two covers what might be considered ethical treatments for "Gender Dysphoria." Part Three covers thoughts from a Catholic perspective on "Gender Dysphoria."

PART ONE

IS "GENDER DYSPHORIA"[1] A MENTAL DISORDER?

Abstract

This is the first of three-parts in this book on the topic of "Gender Dysphoria." This part represents my scientific analysis of this subject based on extensive review of the psychological, psychiatric, and medical literature, consisting of approximately 275 technical papers and many popular articles. The resulting analysis shows the failure of the APA, AMA, AAP, and WHO among others to serve their patient populations. The review examined claims of brain sexual dimorphism and plasticity, variability in the human species, and more. After arguments from mathematics, biological sciences, nature and survival of the species, psychiatric co-morbidities, similarity to other mental disorders, suicidality, ineffectiveness of sex "reassignment" surgeries,[2] and the deficiencies of standards development, the only

---

[1] I will capitalize the term "Gender Dysphoria" and put it in quotation marks in this book unless it is used in a direct quote. In that case, I will follow the style of the paper being cited. The use of quotation marks is meant to highlight the fact that this term was invented to give the impression that the symptoms associated with "Gender Dysphoria" do not define a mental disorder. This will be discussed in more detail throughout this book.

[2] In this book, surgical modification of the body used to affirm gender transitions will be cited as 'sex "reassignment" surgery,' with the word "reassignment" in quotation marks, or I will use "SRS," also in quotes. The purpose in doing so is to emphasize the fact that no matter what pro-

1

logical conclusion is that the symptoms of the phenomenon known to the public as "Gender Dysphoria" do indeed constitute a mental disorder. A series of actions are proposed to address the current societal upheaval being caused by this phenomenon.

Introduction

Although "Gender Dysphoria" is discussed regularly in the popular press and news media, most people don't have an understanding or have never been exposed to the elements which make up the diagnosis in the field of psychiatry and psychology. Therefore, some basic discussion of the terminology and diagnostic criteria is warranted before delving into the technical literature about this phenomenon.

There are individuals in society who experience confusion between their biological sex, and how they mentally perceive themselves. "Gender Dysphoria" is the current overarching term for this confusion, <u>when accompanied by clinically significant distress</u>, according to the American Psychiatric Association (APA). That term, in fact, is the title of a chapter in the Diagnostic and Statistical Man-

---

cedures are done, as discussed later in the book, the biological sex of a person cannot be changed. The only effect of hormone treatments and surgery is to change the appearance of a person to look as if they are members of the opposite sex. According to the principles of biology, it is impossible to change the composition of every cell in the body to render a change in sex of the individual whose body is being considered.

ual of Mental Disorders (5th Ed.)[3] and DSM-5-TR[4] (APA, 2013 and 2022, resp.). The chapter deals with individuals who are not comfortable with the physical sex that was recognized at the time of birth and who experience distress because of that. The APA describes a person's 'physical sex' as the "*gender*" that was "*assigned to them at birth.*"

The DSM is "*a classification of mental disorders with associated criteria designed to facilitate more reliable diagnoses of these disorders. (APA, 2013)*"

Definitions

Some definitions from that manual will be useful in grounding the reader who may be unfamiliar with this topic. All the definitions that follow are taken verbatim from DSM-5[5]:

- "*Gender assignment refers to the initial assignment as male or female. This occurs usually at birth and, thereby, yields the "natal gender."*
- "*Gender identity is a category of social identity and refers to an individual's identification as male, female, or, occasionally, some category other than male or female.*"

---

[3] American Psychiatric Association, *Diagnostic and statistical manual of mental disorders* (5th ed.) (2013) https://doi.org/10.1176/appi.books. 9780890425596

[4] American Psychiatric Association. *Diagnostic and statistical manual of mental disorders* (5th ed., text rev.). (2022). https://doi.org/10.1176/ appi.books.9780890425787

[5] APA, DSM-5, 451.

- "<u>Gender dysphoria</u> *as a general descriptive term refers to an individual's affective/cognitive discontent with the assigned gender..."*

  - "*Gender Dysphoria refers to the **distress** [my emphasis] that may accompany the incongruence between one's experienced or expressed gender and one's assigned gender*"
  - "*The current term is more descriptive than the previous DSM-IV term 'gender identity disorder' and focuses on dysphoria as the clinical problem, not identity per se.*"

- "<u>Transgender</u> *refers to the broad spectrum of individuals who transiently or persistently identify with a gender different from their natal gender.*"
- "<u>Transsexual</u> *denotes an individual who seeks, or has undergone, a social transition from male to female or female to male, which in many, but not all, cases also involves a somatic transition by cross-sex hormone treatment and genital surgery (sex reassignment surgery).*"
- "<u>Gender reassignment</u> *denotes an official (and usually legal) change of gender.*"

As others have done, quoting from Meyer-Bahlburg, in this article, I will use "*'sex' to refer to the congenital somatic and physiolo-*

gical aspects, and 'gender' to denote the behavioral, psychological, and social aspects" of the human.[6]

"Gender Dysphoria," per se, was not included in the first two DSMs - DSM and DSM-II (APA, 1952[7] and APA, 1968[8], reps.), but was included under Sexual Deviations (e.g., Homosexuality or Transvestism). In fact, when the concept of a person uncomfortable with their biological sex was first included in DSM-III, it was called **Gender Identity Disorder (GID)**.[9] *"Across all versions of the DSM since DSM-III, the core construct of GID is the combination of identification with the other gender and of a sense of inappropriateness, if not rejection, of one's assignment to the natal gender...".*[10] [11]

There have been seven versions of the DSM since the original in 1952. These include DSM-II, DSM-III, DSM-III-R, DSM-IV, DSM-IV-TR, DSM-5, and DSM-5-TR. (APA, 1968, 1980, 1987, 1994,

---

[6] Heino F. L Meyer-Bahlburg, "From Mental Disorder to Iatrogenic Hypogonadism: Dilemmas in Conceptualizing Gender Identity Variants as Psychiatric Conditions." *Archives of Sexual Behavior* 39.2 (2010): 461-76.

[7] American Psychiatric Association, *Diagnostic and statistical manual of mental disorders* (APA, 1952), 38-39.

[8] American Psychiatric Association, *Diagnostic and statistical manual of mental disorders,* 2nd ed. (APA, 1968), 44.

[9] American Psychiatric Association, *Diagnostic and statistical manual of mental disorders,* 3rd ed. (APA, 1980), 261.

[10] Meyer-Bahlburg, "From Mental Disorder to Iatrogenic Hypogonadism," 461.

[11] Titia F. Beek, Peggy T. Cohen-Kettenis and Baudewijntje P.C. Kreukels, "Gender incongruence/gender dysphoria and its classification history," *International Review of Psychiatry,* (November 19, 2015): 5-12, online: http://dx.doi.org/10.3109/09540261.2015.1091293

2000, 2013, 2022).[12] During this time, the psychiatric field has undergone intense debate as to whether GID is, in fact, truly a psychiatric <u>disorder</u> or just a "<u>natural variation</u>."

In fact, Vance et al.[13], along with five members of the APA "Sexual and Gender Identity Disorders Working Group," published the results of a survey of *"201 organizations concerned with the welfare of transgender people."* Their quest was to determine opinions from the people in those organizations about various issues with the Gender Identity Disorder diagnosis in DSM-IV. Most of the 'organizations' surveyed (81%) were not mental health professionals but appear to have been advocacy groups for the Transgender and LGBT community (Vance, et al., Table 2)[14]. Only 5 of the 43 groups were *"medical/mental health professionals."* Not surprisingly more than half of the groups (55.8%) wanted GID removed from the next DSM. The main reasons were:

- *"the mere existence of the GID diagnosis is stigmatizing, as it marginalizes individuals who do not conform to the traditional binary construct of gender based on natal sex characteristics"*
- it *"suggests that individuals with GID are sexually deviant"*

---

[12] American Psychiatric Association, *Diagnostic and statistical manual of mental disorders* (2nd, 3rd, 3rd Revised, 4th, 4th Text Revised, 5th, and 5th Text Revised eds.) (APA, 1968, 1980, 1987, 1994, 2000, 2013, 2022).

[13] Stanley R. Vance, Jr., et al., "Opinions About the DSM Gender Identity Disorder Diagnosis: Results from an International Survey Administered to Organizations Concerned with the Welfare of Transgender People," *International Journal of Transgenderism*, 12 (2010): 1–14.

[14] Ibid.

- *"the label "mental disorder" is inherently pejorative, providing an institutionally supported term for use as a discriminatory instrument."[15]*

And the main reason given by the 21% of the groups who said it should remain (Vance, et al., Table 4), was so that sex "reassignment" surgery (sometimes referred to as "SRS" unless inside a quotation), hormonal therapy, and psychotherapy could be reimbursed by insurance companies.[16]

Since that time, and with the publication of DSM-5, there has been a seismic shift in the tone of the DSM.[17] The term *"Gender Dysphoria"* has replaced *"Gender Identity Disorder"* so as not to offend anyone or stigmatize those with gender ambivalence. For example, *"… a governmental agency made Sweden the first country to remove the GIDC diagnosis* [**GIDC is GID in Children**] *from the Swedish version of the ICD-10, citing its potential, along with five other diagnoses, of being offensive and contributing to prejudice."*[18] Similarly the classification of transgender individuals as "mentally ill" was removed[19] in 2011 by the European Parliament and in 2017 by the

---

[15] Ibid.

[16] Ibid.

[17] APA, DSM-5, 451.

[18] Jack Drescher, "Queer Diagnoses: Parallels and Contrasts in the History of Homosexuality, Gender Variance, and the Diagnostic and Statistical Manual." *Archives of Sexual Behavior* 39.2 (2010): 427-60.

[19] Francine Russo, "Where Transgender is No Longer a Diagnosis," *Scientific American*, January 6, 2017. https://www.scientificamerican.com/article/where-transgender-is-no-longer-a-diagnosis/

Danish parliament."[20] And in 2019, the World Health Organization similarly removed Gender Identity Disorder from the list of mental illnesses in the ICD-11 (International Classification of Diseases).[21]

To orient the non-specialist reader, Cohen-Kettenis and Pfäfflin[22] summarized the kernel of all the Gender Identity Disorder diagnoses as "*...the core criteria for transsexualism or GID have always consisted of combinations of the following elements...:*

1. *Cross-gender identification*
2. *Desire to live as a member of the other sex*
3. *Sense of inappropriateness in the gender role belonging to one's natal sex*
4. *Discomfort about one's assigned sex*
5. *Desire to have sex characteristics of the other sex*
6. *Discomfort about one's anatomic sex*
7. *Wish to get rid of one's natal sex characteristics*"

DSM-5 and subsequent editions include a second major criterion, viz. that "**the condition is associated with clinically signifi-**

---

[20] Jack Drescher, Peggy Cohen-Kettenis, and Sam Winter, "Minding the body: Situating gender identity diagnoses in the ICD-11," *International Review of Psychiatry*, 24.6 (December 2012): 568–577.

[21] Dorothy Cummings McLean, "World Health Organization removes Gender Identity Disorder from list of mental illnesses," *Life Site News*, https://www.lifesitenews.com/news/world-health-organization-removes-gender-identity-disorder-from-list-of-mental-illnesses/

[22] Peggy T. Cohen-Kettenis and Friedemann Pfäfflin. "The DSM Diagnostic Criteria for Gender Identity Disorder in Adolescents and Adults." *Archives of Sexual Behavior* 39.2 (2010): 499-513.

cant distress or impairment…" (This was also part of the DSM-IV criteria for GID, but in DSM-5 and following, it is broken out into a necessary criterion in addition to at least six of the above for children or two of the above for adults.)[23] In fact, **it's the distress** that DSM-5 calls the disorder, **not the incongruence** with one's actual physical sex. There will be more about this later.

In this book I will include information about "Gender Dysphoria" in both adults and children (formerly called, GID and GIDC).[24] The rationale for presenting both is that, although there are differences in diagnostic criteria for adults and children, many of the symptoms and criteria are in fact, very similar, if not identical. It appears reasonable to assume that if psychological or biological processes are responsible for the symptoms, they may have the same origins or causes. It should be noted that GIDC includes children who experience discomfort with their biological sex, not those who

---

[23] APA, *DSM-5* and *DSM-5-TR*.

[24] *Caveat Emptor* – As the author of this book, I have no formal degree in psychology or psychiatry. I have a PhD in Physics with a specialty in Biophysics/Biomechanics. I also have bachelor's level training in Religious Studies, and master's level training in Pastoral Studies which includes much study of scripture and some study on the nature of psychological and spiritual development of the human person. Like any research study, this work began with an extensive review of the literature, in this case, scientific, medical, and psychiatric/psychological literature. That review formed the basis for this book which examines views in the literature as to whether "Gender Dysphoria" is a mental disorder. I have focused on that topic because it is central to the entire conclusion that the psychiatric profession has failed its patients. I have attempted to provide a balanced and fair scientific analysis, and to draw conclusions based on logical interpretation of the more than 275 related publications reviewed from literature searches in 2015, 2023, 2024, and 2025.

are uncomfortable with their role as described by their gender (a la Bartlett et al[25]). There is support for this approach from Zucker, who said "*…it was argued that GID in childhood versus adolescence and adulthood were, in effect, the same condition, but expressed differently as a function of developmental level.*" And later, "*… there is no compelling reason to contest in toto the relation between GID in childhood versus adolescence and adulthood.*" [26]

In deference to those experiencing these feelings, I will generally use the terms "Gender Dysphoria" to refer to the feeling experienced by those who are uncomfortable with their anatomic sex (referred to as 'natal gender' by the APA) unless using a direct quote.

Do the Symptoms of "Gender Dysphoria" Constitute a Mental Disorder?

A Review of the Literature

The reasons for the evolutions of the aforementioned diagnostic criteria in the DSMs are many, but they all boil down to a large-scale debate within the field of psychiatry as to whether feeling conflicted with one's anatomic sex is truly a mental disorder. There have been many different proposals for the overarching term indicative of transgender individuals. These include among others: "Gender

---

[25] Nancy H. Bartlett, et al. "Is Gender Identity Disorder in Children a Mental Disorder?", *Sex Roles* 43.11-12 (2000): 753-85.

[26] Kenneth J. Zucker, "The DSM Diagnostic Criteria for Gender Identity Disorder in Children," *Archives of Sexual Behavior* 39.2 (2009): 477-98.

Identity Disorder (GID),"[27] "Atypical Gender Identity Organiza-tion,"[28] "Gender Nonconforming,"[29] "Gender Variant,"[30] "Gender Dysphoria."[31] These terms are the result of the ongoing debate, the fact that the cause of the symptoms is unknown, and the attempt to reduce the stigma to those experiencing this condition.

There is a plethora of studies on this topic and reviewing them all would require several books. A number of studies published mostly over the last two decades are reviewed very briefly here to give the reader an idea of the issues.

John Money was a psychologist who, in the 1950s, developed theories regarding what was called gender identity development (as cited in Drescher[32]). He hypothesized that whether a person consid-ered themselves male or female was not innate or determined by bi-ology but rather was determined by societal and environmental fac-tors. **He also believed that gender identity, once formed, is impos-sible to change.**

Bleiberg, Jackson, and Ross concluded that "*object loss* [(early childhood loss of a parent or important attachment figure)] *and the associated experiences of helplessness and vulnerability*" were impor-

---

[27] APA, *DSM-III.*

[28] Domenico Di Ceglie, "Gender Identity Disorder in Young People," *Advances in Psychiatric Treatment* 6 (2000): 458-66.

[29] Simon Pickstone-Taylor, "Children with Gender Nonconformity," Journal of American Academy of Child and Adolescent Psychiatry 42.3 (2003): 266.

[30] Edgardo J. Menvielle, et al., "To the beat of a different drummer: the gender-variant child," *Contemporary Pediatrics* 22:2 (2005): 38.

[31] APA, DSM-5, 451.

[32] Drescher, "Queer Diagnoses," 427.

tant determinants in disturbances of gender identity in some children. Further, they stated that these children "...*may respond to psychodynamic treatment not specifically designed to alter their gender role behavior, but to resolve their pathological defenses...*"[33]

Marantz and Coates compared mothers of boys with and without "Gender Dysphoria". They found that 53% of mothers of boys with "Gender Dysphoria" had Borderline Personality Disorder or symptoms of Depression compared to only 6% of the mothers of boys without "Gender Dysphoria."[34]

Similarly, Di Ceglie[35] noted that in several case studies, the incongruity between sex and gender identity were the result of early age traumas that resolved after treatment by psychologists. In particular, he found that "[in] *a survey of the first 124 cases referred to the GIDS at the Portman Clinic,... the most common associated features were relationship difficulties with parents or [care-givers] (57%), relationship difficulties with peers (52%), depression/misery (42%), family mental health problems (38%), family physical health problems (38%), being the victim of harassment or persecution (33%) and social sensitivity (31%)."* **This observation led to the hypothesis that the gender identity problem is a mental disorder that is related to the trauma caused by parental depression or major physical illness within the patient's family.**

---

[33] Efrain Bleiberg, Linda Jackson, and Jack L. Ross, "Gender Identity Disorder and Object Loss." *Journal of the American Academy of Child Psychiatry* 25.1 (1986): 58-67.

[34] Sonia Marantz and Susan Coates, "Mothers of Boys with Gender Identity Disorder: A Comparison of Matched Controls." *J American Academy Child Adolescent Psychology* 30.2 (1991): 310-15.

[35] Di Ceglie, "Gender Identity Disorder in Young People," 458.

Bartlett et al. took issue with several of the terms in the definition of a mental disorder in DSM-IV, and with some of the criteria for Gender Dysphoria.[36] The definition of a mental disorder in DSM-IV[37] is as follows:

> "[1] In DSM-IV, each of the mental disorders is conceptualized as a clinically significant behavioral or psychological syndrome or pattern... and that is associated with present distress... or disability (i.e., impairment in... important areas of functioning) or with a significantly increased risk of suffering death, pain, disability....
>
> [2] In addition, this syndrome or pattern must not be merely an expectable and culturally sanctioned response to a particular event, for example, the death of a loved one.
>
> [3] Whatever its original cause, it must currently be considered a manifestation of a behavioral, psychological, or biological **dysfunction** in the individual. [**my emphasis**]
>
> [4] Neither deviant behavior (e.g., political, religious, or sexual) nor conflicts that are primarily between the individual and society are mental disorders unless the deviance or conflict is a symptom of a dysfunction in the individual, as described above" (DSM-IV, pp. xxi, xxii)."

They state that the term **dysfunction** is open to interpretation. One interpretation as cited from Wakefield refers to "*failure of a*

---

[36] Bartlett, et al. "Is Gender Identity Disorder in Children a Mental Disorder?", 753.

[37] APA, *DSM-IV.*

mechanism in a person to perform a natural function for which the mechanism was designed by natural selection."[38]

Bartlett et al. are critical of this definition citing a *"misapplication of evolutionary concepts.* "They also took issue with the apparent confusion of 'sex' and 'gender' in the diagnostic criteria, pointing out that the "...*items in Criterion B are ... problematic because of the confusion of sex and gender. Discomfort with one's biological sex and discomfort with the gender roles ascribed to this category are very different phenomena.*"[39]

Finally, they cited a study by Coates and Person[40] which assessed social and school competence of boys in the 12-14 age range who met the DSM-III criteria for GID. In that study, using the Child Behavior Checklist (CBCL), 80% of the boys scored in the clinical range. What that means is that the behavioral or emotional problems exhibited by the boys were significantly more severe than typical boys of the same age.

Similarly for girls, *"the evidence seems to point to the existence of disability only among those children who experience discomfort with their biological sex."* So, children who behave in ways not typical for their sex (cross-gender behavior, e.g., a boy playing with dolls) do not show signs of disability, but those who have a stated preference

---

[38] J.C. Wakefield, J. C. "Limits of operationalization: A critique of Spitzer and Endicott's (1978) proposed operational criteria for mental disorder," *Journal of Abnormal Psychology*, 102.1 (February 1993): 160–172.

[39] Bartlett, et al. "Is Gender Identity Disorder in Children a Mental Disorder?", 753.

[40] Susan Coates and Ethel Spector Person, "Extreme Boyhood Femininity: Isolated Behavior or Pervasive Disorder?", *Journal of the American Academy of Child Psychiatry* 24:6 (November 1985): 702-709.

to be the other sex do score in the clinical range of the CBCL. This led Bartlett et al. to conclude, among other things, that children *"...who experience discomfort with their biological sex may meet some of the DSM-IV criteria for mental disorder."*

Egan and Perry, in a study of 182 children from 4th through 8th grades (81 M, 101F), found that "[by] *the age of 2 or 3 years, most children can answer correctly the question 'Are you a boy or a girl?'"* and "[by] *age 6 or 7, nearly all children attain full gender constancy..."* In addition, *"...there is considerable variability among persons of a given sex as to the particular constellation of gender-congruent attributes a person displays."* Given this, *"...most people most of the time are able to identify a sufficient amount of gender-congruent attributes to feel comfortably gender typical."*[41]

They further point to the multidimensional aspects of gender identity, and note that *"...by middle childhood, children have developed fairly stable conceptions of (a) the degree to which they typify their gender category, (b) their contentedness with their gender assignment..."*

Diamond holds that gender identity in males is formed during the separation-individuation process in childhood and that gender identity begins with the child's ability to identify with both parents simultaneously.[42] He proposes that the extent to which the gender

---

[41] Susan K. Egan, and David G. Perry, "Gender Identity: A Multidimensional Analysis With Implications For Psychosocial Adjustment." *Developmental Psychology* 37.4 (2001): 451-63.

[42] Michael J. Diamond, "The Shaping of Masculinity: Revisioning Boys Turning Away from Their Mothers to Construct Male Gender Identity." *International Journal of Psychoanalysis* 85 (2004): 359-80.

identity is healthy depends on the interpersonal dynamic between mother and son, and "*…whether there is an available pre-oedipal father.*"[43]

Sisk and Zehr considered the timing of puberty ("*individual becomes capable of sexually reproducing*") with respect to adolescence ("*acquisition of adult cognition, decision making strategies, and social behaviors*") in young humans.[44] They proposed that a linkage exists between puberty and adolescence because the brain is a target for hormones. Depending on the phase of these two developmental cycles, they expect "*individual differences in adult behavior and risk for sex-biased psychopathologies.*" They also noted that there is a link between early puberty and many psychopathologies, such as eating disorders and depression.

Zucker and Spitzer argued that in DSM-III, "*…GIDC was included as a psychiatric diagnosis because it met the generally accepted criteria used by the framers of DSM-III for inclusion (for example, clinical utility…*" and "*…was guided by the reliance on 'expert consensus'…*" Thus, Gender Identity Disorder in Children (along with Transsexualism, and Gender Identity Disorder of Adolescence and Adulthood of a Non-Transsexual type) <u>was considered to be a mental disorder by the experts who made up the DSM-III subcommittee on psychosexual disorders.</u>[45]

---

[43] A "pre-oedipal father" means a father figure in the life of a child between birth and around the age of 3.

[44] Cheryl L. Sisk and Julia L. Zehr, "Pubertal Hormones Organize The Adolescent Brain And Behavior." *Frontiers in Neuroendocrinology* 26 (2005): 163-74.

[45] Kenneth J. Zucker, and Robert L. Spitzer. "Was The Gender Identity Disorder Of Childhood Diagnosis Introduced Into DSM-III As A

Zucker reviewed the diagnostic criteria for Gender Identity Disorder in Children as formulated for DSM-III, DSM-III-R, and DSM-IV.[46] While his article focused on children, it also has some important insights with respect to adolescents and adults with "Gender Dysphoria."

He noted that "[critics] *who reject the GID diagnosis [as a mental disorder] in toto have adopted alternative language to label children who display various degrees of cross-gender behavior and identity. One such label is to... characterize them as 'gender variant'... (Lev, 2004)*" He then provided several definitions from The Oxford Dictionary:

1. Variant - a form or version that varies from other forms of the same thing.'
2. Variation - a change or slight difference in condition, amount, or level.'
3. Variance - the amount by which something changes or is different from something else.'

He pointed out that by these definitions "*...it is descriptively accurate to characterize children who meet the GID criteria as they are currently formulated as gender-variant...*" However, he noted that "[the] *deeper philosophical ... debate is whether or not one can demarcate a distinction between variance and disorder.*" **This question is vital to the considerations at hand.**

Backdoor Maneuver To Replace Homosexuality? A Historical Note." *Journal of Sex & Marital Therapy* 31 (2005): 31-42.

[46] Zucker, "The DSM Diagnostic Criteria for Gender Identity," 477.

Zucker further noted that distress and impairment were used to develop the definition of a mental disorder in the DSM-III to help discern between what is a 'disorder' and what is a 'variation' from the norm. The "clinical significance criterion" of DSM-IV was then based on these concepts. He opined that the best understanding of 'distress' would be given by "*a child's verbalized sense of unhappiness about being a boy or a girl, as expressed most concretely by remarks about wanting to be of the other sex.*"

Zucker pointed out that many qualifiers are used to characterize "Gender Dysphoria," including: *'repeatedly,' 'insistence,' 'strong and persistent,' 'intense,' 'strong,' 'marked,'* among others. He was not sure why all those different terms were used and that there was no consensus on one. He remarked that the subjectivity and imprecision of these labels hampered the reliability of clinical assessments.

Cohen-Kettenis and Pfäfflin argued that "[the] *DSM has consistently approached gender problems from the position that a divergence between the assigned sex... and 'the' psychological sex (gender) per se signals a psychiatric disorder.*"[47] However, they note that most of the publications on "Gender Dysphoria" have ignored the severity of the condition. They appear to be advocating allowing for the diagnosis of psychiatric disorder only in more severe cases of gender conflicts.

Levine and Solomon, as cited in Drescher,[48] proffered that Gender Identity Disorders "*...are forms of psychopathology,*" and "*...are*

---

[47] Cohen-Kettenis, and Pfäfflin. "The DSM Diagnostic Criteria for Gender Identity, 499.

[48] Stephen B. Levine and Anna Solomon, "Meanings and Political Implications of "Psychopathology" in a Gender Identity Clinic: A Report of

typically co-morbid with other psychopathologies." They considered the "*promotion of civil rights for the transgendered* [to have obscured] *professional perceptions of psychopathology.*" They also made it clear that there is much uncertainty "*...about the long-term outcome of gender transition and sex reassignment surgery.*"

They offer that the three advantages of considering "Gender Dysphoria" as a mental disorder are 1) it is more likely to be studied scientifically, 2) medical insurers are more likely to pay for evaluation and therapy, and 3) some of the suffering of these patients may be treatable.

Drescher compared the debate about whether "Gender Dysphoria" is a mental disorder to a similar debate that took place decades earlier about homosexuality. He noted that "[the]... *APA's scientific body addressing this issue, also wrestled with the question of what constitutes a mental disorder. Spitzer (1981), who chaired a subcommittee..., 'reviewed the characteristics of the various mental disorders and concluded that... they all regularly caused subjective distress or were associated with generalized impairment in social effectiveness'.*"[49]

Drescher was very critical of the paper by Levine and Solomon saying that there are "*...obvious narrative contradictions of their approach.*" He also recommended separation of the diagnosis of "Gender Dysphoria" in Children from "Gender Dysphoria" in adults. He considered etiologic links between the two to be unfounded. He wondered whether there are subtypes of "Gender Identity Disorder"

---

10 Cases." *Journal of Sex & Marital Therapy* 35.1 (2008): 40-57 as cited in Drescher, "Queer Diagnoses," 427.

[49] Ibid.

in children because, **as he pointed out, most cases in children resolve themselves before they become adults.**

His discussion of the philosophical dimensions of the debate is
worth repeating at some length. He noted that "[subjective] *considerations were not entirely lost on the architect of the current DSM diagnostic system, Robert Spitzer (1981), who struggled with similar
questions decades ago.*" Spitzer claimed that "[the] *concept of disorder is man-made,* [and that over] *the course of time, all cultures have
evolved concepts of illness or disease in order to identify certain conditions that, because of their negative consequences, implicitly have a
call to action...*"

"*Spitzer, charged with answering the question of whether homosexuality should be considered a psychiatric diagnosis, came up with
a unique formulation: psychiatric disorders are characterized by dysfunction and distress... In DSM-III each of the mental disorders is
conceptualized as a clinically significant behavioral or psychological
syndrome or pattern that occurs in an individual and that is typically
associated with either a painful symptom (distress) or impairment in
one or more important areas of functioning (disability). In addition,
there is an inference that there is a behavioral, psychological, or biological dysfunction, and that the disturbance is not only in the relationship between the individual and society.*"

Meyer-Bahlburg compared developmental similarities between
homosexuality and "Gender Dysphoria." He noted that both sexual
orientation and gender identity are exhibited in a spectrum of behaviors, and that homosexuality can also be viewed as a gender-

atypical behavior.[50] In addition, "...*both homosexuals and people with GIVs* [Gender Identity Variations] *suffer extensive societal stigma and, probably in part as a consequence, increased psychiatric problems, although bidirectional causation cannot be ruled out.*"

In a discussion of etiology, Meyer-Bahlburg noted that various authors have found "*increased psychiatric problems in the parents of children with GIV*" and that "...*familiality and heritability are common findings in psychiatric conditions.*"

In searching for a way to determine whether GIV is a disorder, Meyer-Bahlburg also consulted the dictionary. "*In general, the demarcation of behaviors that are 'pathologic' from those that are not poses a challenge to the clinician. Stedman's Medical Dictionary (1995) defines 'pathology' as the 'medical science, and specialty practice, concerned with all aspects of disease, but with special reference to the essential nature, causes, and development of abnormal conditions...' Yet, the Stedman definition of pathology obviously presupposes a consensus on the definition of 'disease,' and does not offer a systematic approach to demarcate psychopathologic from non-psychopathologic*"

He noted that "...*part of the categorization problem is due to the fact that we do not have a well-established detailed theory - let alone a neuroanatomic / neurophysiologic model - of normal gender identity development that [helps distinguish] non-pathologic from pathologic. Under these circumstances, causal directions among psychological processes are notoriously difficult to establish, which makes the*

---

[50] Meyer-Bahlburg, "From Mental Disorder to Iatrogenic Hypogonadism," 461.

delineation of pathologic processes problematic." So, clear criteria to differentiate normal from pathologic gender identity development are not available. Furthermore, in clinical practice, the distress and impairment criteria are not always applicable.

Relative to "Gender Dysphoria in Children" vs "Gender Dysphoria in Adults," he denies that the separation of child and adolescent or adult GIVs is warranted from either a scientific or clinical basis. Further, even though the number of cases that resolve themselves is higher in young children than in adults, "*the difference is only a matter of degree and diminishes with age.*"

Meyer-Bahlburg concluded that "*In the absence of an empirically grounded detailed theory of the mechanisms and processes of gender identity development, the available empirical evidence does not permit a categorical, universally valid statement that GIVs are or are not mental disorders.*"

Along these lines, in the landmark study by the U.S. Department of Health and Human Services on pediatric "Gender Dysphoria," the authors note, "*the diagnostic criteria for GD are based solely on subjective reports and behavioral observations in patients with no objective physical pathology; there are no verifiable physiological or biochemical markers—such as abnormal imaging, lab, or clinical findings—to confirm the GD diagnosis.*"[51]

Rajkumar analyzed the rates of schizophrenia and "Gender Dysphoria" in the population and compared those to the rates of co-

---

[51] U.S. Department of Health and Human Services (hereafter, HHS), "Treatment for Pediatric Gender Dysphoria - Review of Evidence and Best Practices" (2025) https://opa.hhs.gov/gender-dysphoria-report.

occurrence of the two conditions.[52] He notes that "[a] *relationship between two distinct disorders can be inferred if they cooccur at a higher level than would be expected by chance.*" His data that shows co-occurrence between schizophrenia and "Gender Dysphoria" should only be seen in 1 in 1,000,000 individuals. However, rates in published studies appear to be much greater than that and greater that the rate of schizophrenia in the general population. He posits a common neurodevelopmental disorder as the cause of both.

Finally, Colizzi et al. studied 118 patients with "Gender Dysphoria." Nearly half 45.8% reported childhood trauma in the form of abuse and/or neglect, suggesting that it could "*have a role...in the development of gender identity.*" [53] Still, even with all of the aforementioned research, they noted that "*the origins of gender dysphoria are still largely unclear.*"

As noted earlier, DSM-5 states that "Gender Dysphoria" refers to the state of mind of an individual who is not happy with their "assigned" gender.[54] Specifically, "*Gender Dysphoria refers to the distress that may accompany the incongruence between one's experi-*

---

[52] Ravi Philip Rajkumar, "Gender Identity Disorder and Schizophrenia: Neurodevelopmental Disorders with Common Causal Mechanisms?" *Schizophrenia Research and Treatment* (2014): 1-8, Article ID 463757, http://dx.doi.org/10.1155/2014/463757.

[53] Marco Colizzi, Rosalia Costa, and Orlando Todarello. "Dissociative Symptoms in Individuals with Gender Dysphoria: Is the Elevated Prevalence Real?" *Psychiatry Research In Press* (2015): 173-80.

[54] Note that I have placed "assigned" in quotation marks to bring to mind the fact that a person's sex at birth is not "assigned," but is a biological fact. In this context, it will always be in quotes unless part of a cited quotation.

enced or expressed gender and one's assigned gender. Although not all individuals will experience distress as a result of such incongruence, many are distressed if the desired physical interventions by means of hormones and/or surgery are not available." [55] DSM-5 concentrates on the dysphoria as the problem, not the identity confusion.

The HHS study notes that this shifting of emphasis with respect to "Gender Dysphoria" was a result of the *"tension between ensuring reimbursement and thereby access, on the one hand, and satisfying the demands of patients and activist groups for depathologization, on the other..."* [56] This shift resulted in the DSM declaring that *"experiencing gender incongruence itself is not pathological, while associated distress or impairment* [is]." [57]

Does Sexual Dimorphism in the Brain Mean "Gender Dysphoria" is not a Mental Disorder?

For the past 20 plus years there has been a desperate search using brain imaging techniques to show that people with "Gender Dysphoria" have brains, or more appropriately, have some brain structures, that resemble the brains/structures opposite their natal sex. This is usually associated with the term "sexual dimorphism." As the Greek root *"morphe"* implies, sexual dimorphism is the concept that male brains and/or brain structures are different in shape and or size from female brains and/or brain structures. In particular, this research aims to show that the brains of people with "Gender Dysphoria" are

---

[55] APA, DSM-5, 451.

[56] HHS, "Treatment for Pediatric Gender Dysphoria," 229.

[57] HHS, "Treatment for Pediatric Gender Dysphoria," 230.

more like the brains of their "experienced gender" than their "natal gender" (sex).

During my first review of the literature, I found study after study claiming to prove this hypothesis. However, every study had some critical issue that made the claim doubtful at best. Most of the studies had very small numbers of subjects. This is important because, as much as we are all similar in some respects, there is amazing variability in the human species.

Meyer-Bahlburg noted that while there has been much ado about recent anatomic findings, they have also been associated with *"...large within-group variability and cross-group overlap."* [58] And not many of the findings have been replicated or even explained, so that it is difficult to make a pronouncement based on the available evidence.

In a large-scale meta-analysis of asymmetry in the subcortical human brain, Guadalupe et al.[59] examined Asymmetry Indices (AI) of substructures in the human brain within a dataset of 15,847 human subject MRIs from 52 datasets worldwide. They observed different means across the datasets indicating that measurements on many brain structures are susceptible to methodological biases. They note that their study "__underlines__ *the utility, and indeed* __the necessity__ *of analyzing subtle subcortical asymmetries in* __vast samples__

---

[58] Meyer-Bahlburg, "From Mental Disorder to Iatrogenic Hypogonadism," 461.

[59] Tulio Guadalupe, Samuel R. Mathias, Theo G.M. vanErp, et al. "Human subcortical brain asymmetries in 15,847 people worldwide reveal effects of age and sex," *Brain Imaging and Behavior* 11 (2017): 1497–1514, DOI 10.1007/s11682-016-9629-z.

(my emphases)." They also noted a "*significant* [non-linear] *effect of age on the AI*" of at least one brain structure, meaning that studies which do not control for age could be in serious error.

Similarly, Byne et al.[60] state, "*while some positive findings in the predicted direction have been reported, inferences are currently limited. This is because few findings have been replicated and few studies have adequately controlled for potentially confounding variables such as age, sexual orientation, transition status (including history of gender-affirming hormonal treatment, if any), and hormonal status at the time of study (or of death in the case of postmortem studies).*"

In statistics there is an important concept known as "statistical power." Statistical power is related to the ability to detect significant differences among samples of the population. As the population variance increases, the number of samples needed to accurately detect differences between samples increases. That is, the more diverse a population, the less statistical power.

Two distributions with large overlap have low statistical power and therefore require much larger sample sizes to determine significance. Similarly, even if there is a statistical significance between means, the size of the effect as measured by "Cohen's d" is important. Typically, only when Cohen's d $>= 0.80$ are the differences meaningful. As a rule of thumb, the number of samples needed for a study to be able to determine significant differences is: $n = 16 * (s^2/d^2)$, where s is an estimate of the population variance and d is the difference to

---

[60] William Byne Dan H. Karasic, Eli Coleman, et al. "Gender dysphoria in adults: an overview and primer for psychiatrists," *Transgender Health* 3:1 (2018) 57–A3, DOI: 10.1089/trgh.2017.0053.

be detected. So, as the population variance increases, the number of samples rises as the variance squared! Similarly, as the difference to be detected decreases, the number of samples increases as the inverse of the size squared! So, the small sample sizes of the published studies are very problematic.

It makes sense to seek an organic, chemical, or physical cause for mental illness. After all most of society behaves one way and people with mental illness behave in a very different way. There must be some reason for that, some cause to have an effect like that. The search for differences in brain anatomical structures is in part a search for scientific knowledge. It can also be viewed as a way to "prove" that "Gender Dysphoria" is physical in origin as if that means it is not a mental disorder. Another rationale may be to be able to say, "I was born this way." Do either of these points really matter? No reasonable person would blame a patient with "Gender Dysphoria" for their illness any more than blaming a person with cerebral palsy, or with any number of pathological conditions recognized at birth, for their condition. The fact is, with respect to whether or not "Gender Dysphoria" is a mental disorder, it doesn't matter whether it was present at birth or whether the patient has different organ sizes within the brain. Such knowledge may help understand the phenomenon better and may even enable pharmacological treatments, but both are immaterial to the question at hand.

Variability in the Human Species

There is a spectrum of human behaviors from nurturer to warrior, and each person has some combination of these on the spectrum. That doesn't mean that nurturing men are not men, or tough women are not women. The lay understanding of "Gender Dysphoria" is that the person "feels like a man (woman) trapped in woman's (man's) body." Human beings are born genetically and biologically as male or female (intersex conditions are clearly a different discussion).[61] If a person purports to feel like the other sex, that is objectively delusional because no one can know what it feels like to be another person or gender. What the person may feel is likely what they perceive as the way a man or woman feels based on societal behavioral stereotypes. This feeling defies the objective reality of their given chromosomal make-up.[62] The mind is easily fooled, but chromosomes don't lie. Reality is not defined by our feelings.

After 32 years researching how humans are injured in automotive collisions and designing safety systems to protect them, it is quite clear to me that human beings fall on a vast dimensional spectrum. Just look at the sizes of adult crash test dummies. There is a 95th percentile male, a 50th percentile male, and a 5th percentile female. The sizes, weights, body segment lengths, and circumferences of human beings all vary enormously in the population. For example, the 95th percentile male standing height is 6' 1" tall (186 cm), but the average or 50th percentile male standing height is 5' 9" tall (175 cm), and the

---

[61] Complete and Partial Androgen Insensitivity Syndromes (CAIS and PAIS) along with Intersex conditions (children born with ambiguous genitalia) are separate and complex issues not part of this discussion.

[62] Cara Buskmiller and Paul Hruz, "A Biological Understanding of Man and Woman," in *Sexual Identity: The Harmony of Philosophy, Science, and Revelation*, ed. John Desilva Finley (Steubenville: Emmaus Road, 2022), 70, 75.

5th percentile female is 5'0" (152.8cm). [63] [64] [65] [66] The 5th percentile male, not represented by a crash test dummy, is 5'4" tall (163.6 cm).[67] These values are based on thousands of measurements. To make matters more complicated, these values differ by race and by sex. One reference compiled in 1974 showed that black men had the longest leg lengths, with white men averaging 1.5" (3.8 cm) shorter, and Asian men averaging 3.6" (9.1 cm) shorter than white men.[68]

Similarly, sizes of human organs are shown to vary widely. For example, Luders et al. noted that many neuroanatomical studies on sex differences in brain size, have shown that men have ≈8–10% larger brains than women. *"However, that does not mean that all men have a large brain and all women have small brains. In recent studies we found that ≈15–20% of women have brains of comparable size to men; likewise, ≈15–20% of men had brain sizes similar to those of women."*[69] Similarly, Oberman et al. showed as much as 10% varia-

---

[63] Lawrence W. Schneider, D.H. Robbins, M.A. Pflug, "Anthropometry of Motor Vehicle Occupants (AMVO)." US DOT, NHTSA Contract DTNH22-80-C-07502, Final Report, pg. I-18 and pg. I-10 (respectively), 1983.

[64] Ibid., pg. I-10.

[65] N. Diffrient, A.R. Tilley, and J.C. Bardagjy, *Humanscale* (Cambridge: The MIT Press, 1974), 6.

[66] Human Factors Engineering Technical Advisory Group, *Human Engineering Design Data Digest*, (Washington, DC: Department of Defense, 2000).

[67] Ibid.

[68] N. Diffrient, *Humanscale*, Chart 1a.

[69] Eileen Luders, Helmuth Steinmetz, Lutz Jancke, "Brain size and grey matter volume in the healthy human brain," *Cognitive Neuroscience and Neuropsychology – Neuro Report* 13:17 (2002): 2371-2374.

tion in the diameters of living human hearts based on analysis of X-Rays from 3,985 subjects.[70]

More to the point, Kim et al.[71] reported a study using "*largescale multimodal brain imaging of grey matter morphometric data* [including surface area, mean curvature, thickness, and volume] *and white matter connectomes*" in 9,658 prepubertal children. They used a machine learning model to classify biological sex based on the input shape and connectivity data. The resulting brain-based scores were compared by sex. Geary[72] commented on the results and showed that while most boys have morphometric and connectome patterns that are very similar to each other (concentrated on one side of the brain-based sex score histogram), there is a distribution of lower but finite numbers of boys with brain-based sex scores that span the entire range of brain-based sex scores. In other words, some boys have brains that appear to be like those of girls based on shape and connectivity. So, there is a natural variation in brain features that spans differences in natal sex.

Eliot and co-workers have done landmark retrospective "meta-analyses" of the previously published data that ostensibly showed

---

[70] Albert Oberman, Allen R. Myers, Thomas M. Karunas, Frederick H. Epstein, "Heart Size of Adults in a Natural Population-Tecumseh, Michigan," *Circulation* 35 (1967): 724-733.

[71] Kakyeong Kim et al., "The sexual brain, genes, and cognition: A machine-predicted brain sex score explains individual differences in cognitive intelligence and genetic influence in young children," *Human Brain Mapping* 43 (2022): 3857-3872.

[72] David C. Geary, "The Ideological Refusal to Acknowledge Evolved Sex Differences," *The Quillette* (2022) https://quillette.com/2022/09/01/the-ideological-refusal-to-acknowledge-evolved-sex-differences/

sexual dimorphism of some organs within human brains.[73][74][75][76] Their conclusion was "*Summarizing across the extensive findings we reviewed, [sex/gender] differences in the human brain are extremely subtle and variable. There is nothing to justify the term "sexual dimorphism" to describe them.*" That is, male brains and female brains are essentially the same from an anatomical structural standpoint and the sizes of various organs lie on a distribution with a high degree of overlap.

Among the deficiencies they found in previous studies, very small sample sizes reigned supreme, but also largely a failure to account for differences in total brain volume, lack of control of the methodology including structural segmentation software, normalization algorithms, and choice of normalization standard.

Measurement differences in total brain volume can be corrected by normalizing measurements. Normalization procedures have been used extensively in automotive safety research to develop force-deflection corridors for anthropomorphic test devices (known collo-

---

[73] Lise Eliot, "The Trouble with Sex Differences," *Neuron* 72 (December 22, 2011): 895-898.

[74] Anh Tan, Wenli Ma, Amit Vira, et al., "The human hippocampus is not sexually-dimorphic: Meta-analysis of structural MRI volumes," *NeuroImage* 124 (2016): 350-366.

[75] Dhruv Marwha, Meha Halari, Lise Eliot, "Meta-analysis reveals a lack of sexual dimorphism in human amygdala volume," *NeuroImage* 147 (2017): 282-294.

[76] Lise Eliot, Adnan Ahmed, Hiba Khan, Julie Patel, "Dump the 'dimorphism': Comprehensive synthesis of human brain studies reveals few male-female differences beyond size," *Neuroscience and Biobehavioral Reviews*125 (2021): 667-697.

quially as crash test dummies).[77] These statistical procedures take data from mechanical tests with post-mortem subjects of various sizes and shapes and transform the data so that the force and deflections represent what the subject's response would be if they were all the same size and shape. Then, you are left with the true variation in mechanical response in the sample population.

Given the works of Eliot et al. above, the studies which purport to show that the brains of transgender individuals are more like their perceived gender, are in error. There are currently no studies that reliably demonstrate anatomical differences between the brains of transgender individuals and those who do not report such feelings.

So, do the Symptoms of "Gender Dysphoria" Constitute a Mental Disorder?

A reasonable place to start in answering this question is with another definition of terms. According to Webster's New World Dictionary, the term *"disorder"* means *"a lack of order... confusion... an upset of normal function... [or] disease".*[78] Disorder, implies that there is an "order," or a "norm" or "normal." Again, according to Webster's, the term *"normal"* means conforming with or constituting an accepted standard, model, or pattern; especially, corresponding to the

---

[77] Stephen W. Rouhana, David C. Viano, Edward A. Jedrzejczak, Joseph D. McCleary, "Assessing Submarining and Abdominal Injury Risk in the Hybrid III Family of Dummies," *Stapp Car Crash Journal* 33 (1989): 542-564.

[78] Webster's New World Dictionary, College Edition (New York and Cleveland: World Publishing Co., 1964), 421.

median or average of a large group in type, appearance, achievement, function, development, etc...."[79]

This is the first concept in need of expansion. While society, in general, abhors the term "normal," when applied to individual human beings, the APA itself uses it quite frequently in DSM-5. [80] For example, "Magical thinking may be a part of normal child development," on page 824. In fact, DSM-5 uses the term "normal" and 'abnormal" 13 (thirteen) times in the Glossary on pages 817-831. And the term appears in many places within the rest of DSM-5.

As noted earlier, Gender Identity Disorder was first mentioned in DSM-III in 1980.[81] In subsequent years, researchers and politicians have sought to change the term, so as not to offend anyone (a la Sweden).[82] [83]

Spitzer claimed that the concept of a disorder is man-made.[84] That led him to come up with the formula that in order for symptoms to be indicative of a psychiatric disorder there had to be evidence of **dysfunction** and **distress**. Zucker noted that "[distress] *and impair-*

---

[79] Webster's New World Dictionary, College Edition, 1001.

[80] APA, DSM-5, 451.

[81] APA, *DSM-III*.

[82] Russo, F.: "Where Transgender is No Longer a Diagnosis," *Scientific American*, January 6, 2017, https://www.scientificamerican.com/article/where-transgender-is-no-longer-a-diagnosis/.

[83] Life Site: "World Health Organization removes Gender Identity Disorder from list of mental illnesses," https://www.lifesitenews.com/news/world-health-organization-removes-gender-identity-disorder-from-list-of-mental-illnesse.

[84] Robert L. Spitzer, "The diagnostic status of homosexuality in DSM-III: a reformulation of the issues" *American Journal of Psychiatry* 138:2 (February 1981): 210-215.

ment ... were used to formulate a working definition of mental disorder for the DSM-III... to set some kind of boundary between disorder and variation from the norm..."[85]

Distress has been interpreted by Drescher, for example, as a "*behavioral or psychological syndrome... with... a painful symptom.*"[86] Zucker opined that the best understanding of 'distress' would be given by "*a child's verbalized sense of unhappiness about being a boy or a girl, as expressed most concretely by remarks about wanting to be of the other sex.*"[87] Then, by Spitzer's and Zucker's definitions, any child that persistently expresses a desire to be of the other sex should be considered to have a mental disorder.

Given the suicide rate in those with "Gender Dysphoria," it is clear that their symptoms are psychologically painful and, therefore, are evidence of "distress." The term "disordered" and "normal" are qualitative medical and scientific terms that are meant to be descriptive of a recognizable state of pathology or the freedom from a pathological state. They are not meant to be pejorative or demeaning.

Some argue that it is society that causes the distress. Undoubtedly, there is some truth in that statement. However, it is not all society's doing. People with "Gender Dysphoria" know that they are different, "not normal." To me, it would seem that such self-knowledge itself would be very likely to be the main cause of distress and the main driver for the unfortunately high suicide rate as in other mental disorders. Zucker expresses a similar sentiment, noting

---

[85] Zucker, "The DSM Diagnostic Criteria for Gender Identity," 477.

[86] Drescher, "Queer Diagnoses," 427.

[87] Zucker, "The DSM Diagnostic Criteria for Gender Identity," 477.

that there "*must be in-the-person distress regarding the disjunction between somatic sex and felt psychological gender.*"[88]

One could also argue that only "distress" could lead a person to allow infusion of dangerous chemicals into their bodies or to so mutilate their bodies as to render them incapable of ever naturally bearing children. Again, Zucker expresses a similar sentiment. "*It is difficult to argue that cross-gender feelings and behaviors... do not constitute an example of impairment if one considers the... "end state" of GID... in females: mastectomy, phalloplasty; in males: penectomy/ castration, vaginoplasty... The required physical interventions are simply too radical to be thought about otherwise.*"[89]

While LGBT activists would argue that "Gender Dysphoria" and its "treatment" by hormone replacement therapy and "SRS" does not hurt anyone, it would seem that the person most harmed by these interventions is the patient himself or herself. But it does not stop there, as families are also torn apart when a son or daughter, brother or sister, announces that they are not the person their family has come to know and love, and relationships are redefined.

The term **dysfunction** gets a lot of attention from Bartlett et al.[90] Specifically, they note: "*The issue of whether discomfort with one's biological sex is a dysfunction in the individual is even more problematic. Outright repudiation of one's biological sex certainly seems 'dysfunc-*

---

[88] Kenneth J. Zucker, "Gender Identity Disorder in Children and Adolescents," *Annual Review of Clinical Psychology* 1 (2005): 467–92, DOI: 10.1146/annurev.clinpsy.1.102803.144050.

[89] Ibid.

[90] Bartlett, "Is Gender Identity Disorder in Children a Mental Disorder?" 753.

tional,' at least in the folk sense of the word. However, this sort of intu-
itive 'hunch' is clearly an unacceptable foundation upon which to base
a clinical diagnosis."

Bartlett's statement appears again to indicate a bias on the part of
the authors. Anyone who does not accept reality has a dysfunction.
"Gender Dysphoria" is no different in this sense than Anorexia Nervosa or Body Integrity Identity Disorder, both considered mental
disorders in the DSM. Human beings are born genetically and biologically as males or females. If a person purports to feel like the
other sex, that is objectively delusional because no one can know
what it feels like to be another person or gender, and because it defies
the objective reality of their given chromosomal make-up. Wearing
a dress, for example, and speaking in a high voice, making effeminate
gestures and the like, do not make a man a woman. Men have no idea
what goes on in the minds of women and vice versa. The mind is
easily fooled, but chromosomes don't lie. Reality is not defined by
our feelings.

As Cohen-Kettenis and Pfäfflin pointed out, the core criteria
have changed at least 4 times from DSM-III where they were first
espoused to DSM-IV-TR (their article was written before the prom-
ulgation of DSM-5).[91] This indicates that the psychiatric community
does not have a good understanding of the cause of these issues. It is
often dangerous to treat something without knowing what caused it.
Although this is not unlike much of medicine today where symptoms are often addressed without knowing the underlying reasons
for them. While admittedly, this can bring short-term relief to

---

[91] Cohen-Kettenis, and Pfäfflin, "The DSM Diagnostic Criteria for Gender Identity, 499.

patients; if the underlying causes are not addressed, the ultimate result can be fatal.

The similarities between "Gender Dysphoria" and other psychological disorders also gives pause to those outside of psychiatry looking in. In her paper on Body Integrity Identity Disorder (BIID), Müller[92] cited Furth and Smith[93] who "...*translated the definition of GID 1:1* [one-to-one] *into the definition of BIID*," simply by replacing the words "*male*" and "*female*" with "*able-bodied*" and "*disabled*." BIID is recognized by the DSM as a mental disorder.

All of these disorders have something in common – they are the result of mental disease, possibly of neurochemical, hormonal, or biological origin. Bipolar Disorder and BIID are acknowledged to be mental disorders because it is obvious. To a scientist outside the psychiatric community, "Gender Dysphoria" also seems obvious, but in the present culture of political correctness it seems that any sexual deviation from the norm is assumed to be good and celebrated. Drescher noted earlier that even governments (Sweden in his citation) had gone as far as removing the diagnosis in order not to offend anyone.[94]

In his review of the diagnostic criteria for "GIDC", Zucker noted that critics of the GID diagnosis use the term '**gender variant**' to describe children who display cross-gender behavior and identities,

---

[92] Sabine Muller, "Body Integrity Identity Disorder (BIID) - Is the Amputation of Healthy Limbs Ethically Justified?" *The American Journal of Bioethics* 9:1 (2009): 36-43.

[93] Greg M. Furth and Robert Smith, *Apotemnophilia: Information, Questions, Answers, and Recommendations About Self-Demand Amputation* (Bloomington, IN: 1st Books, 2000).

[94] Drescher, "Queer Diagnoses," 427.

providing several definitions from the Oxford dictionary.[95] He adeptly highlighted the key question in this debate, which is *"whether or not one can demarcate a distinction between variance and disorder."* As pointed out earlier in this manuscript, he also highlighted a difficulty in terminology with respect to the characteristics of the symptoms. His observation that the experts cannot agree upon a single word or phrase to describe the symptoms shows how subjective some diagnoses can be. Children and adults who meet the same criteria should be diagnosed as having the same disorder.

In their survey of 17 "Gender Dysphoria" treatment centers, Vrouenraets et al. noted *"you would not need medical procedures to make the lives of people with gender dysphoria more satisfying if it were merely a normal variation."*[96]

This sentiment was echoed in the more recent HHS publication which observed, *"…a fundamental tension exists between WPATH's desire to treat transgender identity (gender incongruence) as a normal and healthy variation of human development and its insistence that gender incongruence requires "medically necessary" treatment."*[97]

Hence it is important to come back to what variant and disordered mean. Variant and disordered can be defined as being different from the norm. But what is 'normal'? Who is to decide if something is normal and hence what other things are disordered or variant.

---

[95] Zucker, "The DSM Diagnostic Criteria for Gender Identity," 477.

[96] Lieke J. J. Vrouenraets, A. Miranda Fredriks, Sabine E. Hannema, et al. "Early Medical Treatment of Children and Adolescents with Gender Dysphoria: An Empirical Ethical Study." *J Adolescent Health* 57.4 (June 25, 2015): 367-373.

[97] HHS, "Treatment for Pediatric Gender Dysphoria," 189.

Argument from Mathematics

Well, clearly one approach is strictly mathematical. If less than one tenth of one percent (0.1%) of the population behaves in some way, they are clearly not mathematically normal. In fact, they are beyond two standard deviations from the norm, which in most medical cases would certainly imply pathology. Imagine a patient with bone mineral density T score of -3 which is 3 standard deviations worse than the mean or norm. Then, 99.7% of all patients have better bone mineral density. This patient would be considered to have a disease called osteoporosis by any measure.

Argument from Biological Sciences

Mayer and McHugh[98] note that "*[In] biology, an organism is male or female if it is structured to perform one of the respective roles in reproduction.*" They assert that a conceptual basis for biological categories of male and female is found in these reproductive roles. In addition, they stated "*the scientific definition of biological sex is, for almost all human beings, clear, binary, and stable, reflecting an underlying biological reality…*"

Likewise, a position paper on Gender Identity from the American College of Pediatricians published in February of 2024, provided a definitive scientific explanation of the biology of human sex. They stated, "*the sex of an individual is based upon biology and not upon*

---

[98] Lawrence S. Mayer and Paul R. McHugh, "Sexuality and Gender: Findings from the Biological, Psychological, and Social Sciences." *The New Atlantis* 50 (Fall 2016): 10–143.

thoughts or feelings. The individual's sex is encrypted in every diploid cell of the body. Since an individual's biological sex is immutable from the moment of fertilization, it cannot be changed, regardless of hormonal or surgical interventions... [A] *so-called "transition" is not a change of sex or even a change of sexual/gender identity, but rather only a change in sexual appearance or presentation. Thus, "transgender" and "transition" are misleading and inaccurate terms..."*[99]

Similarly, the HHS report states, *"'Assigned sex at birth' is not a harmless euphemism. It suggests an arbitrary decision—not unlike "assigned seating"—rather than the observation of a characteristic present long before birth, namely the child's sex."*[100]

This echoes McHugh[101] who stated, *"Transgendered men do not become women, nor do transgendered women become men. All... become feminized men or masculinized women, counterfeits or impersonators of the sex with which they 'identify.'"*

Argument from Nature and Survival of the Species

Based on Simerly, we are led to a major argument for "Gender Dysphoria" being a disorder. Simerly noted that "[from] *an evolutionary perspective, the most adaptive physiological responses are those that ensure successful reproduction,"* and that *"sex-specific behaviors*

---

[99] American College of Pediatricians, "Mental Health in Adolescents with Incongruence of Gender Identity and Biological Sex," Position Statement, February 2024.

[100] HHS, "Treatment for Pediatric Gender Dysphoria," 32.

[101] Paul R. McHugh, "Transgenderism: A Pathogenic Meme" *Public Discourse*, https://www.thepublicdiscourse.com/2015/06/15145/.

and physiological responses [are] *vital to the success of mammalian species.*"[102]

The HHS report notes that in using estrogen for male medical transitions, "*testicular atrophy results, leading to impaired fertility or infertility that may be irreversible (even if estrogen were to be discontinued).*"[103] Likewise, in sex "reassignment" surgeries, male and female organs of generation are typically removed. Thus, for transgender individuals and, especially for transsexuals, one of the major consequences of "SRS" is that they become incapable of propagating the species. This flies in the face of all evolutionary designs. Then, just based on nature, the symptoms of gender incongruence associated with "Gender Dysphoria" must be a disorder, because its ultimate manifestation leads to complete inability to naturally propagate and continue the species.

Argument from Psychiatric Co-Morbidities

The literature is replete with papers demonstrating that patients with "Gender Dysphoria" are often experiencing many co-existing mental illnesses. The main question which no one has yet been able to answer is whether these co-morbidities are causal (represent the etiology of the disorder), associative (represent a constellation of symptoms of a single, more general disorder), or are caused by the stigma and social ostracism that often accompanies those with

---

[102] Richard B. Simerly, "Wired for Reproduction: Organization and Development of Sexually Dimorphic Circuits in the Mammalian Forebrain." *Annual Review of Neuroscience* 25 (2002): 507-36.

[103] HHS, "Treatment for Pediatric Gender Dysphoria," 115.

"Gender Dysphoria." All **emphasis** in the following section is mine and not from the original authors of the studies cited.

Bradley and Zucker[104] found that "*[rates] of associated psycho-pathology in children with GID are comparable with those in children with other psychiatric disorders, particularly disorders that are inter-nalizing in form.*"

Di Ceglie[105] posited that "*...high percentages of mental and phys-ical health problems <u>in the families</u> of children and adolescents referred may indicate that factors such as parental depression or major physical illness may represent a traumatic event for the child, possibly contrib-uting to the gender identity problem.*"

Bartlett, et al.[106] analyzed "*...the large-scale study of gender-re-ferred boys and girls using the Child Behavior Checklist (CBCL) re-ported by Zucker and Bradley (1995)...*", and found that "*... 62% of gender-referred boys aged 6-11 had sum scores in the clinical range, compared to 29% of male siblings at this age*" and "*...at least 50% scored in the clinical range for Schizoid, Depressed, Uncommunicative, Obsessive-Compulsive, and Social Withdrawal.*" In fact, "*<u>[for] both boys and girls [with GIDC], behavior problem scores exceeded that of the comparison group of siblings</u>.*"

Similarly, Hepp et al. in a study specifically on adult Gender Identity Disordered patients, found that 42% of their subjects had

---

[104] Susan J. Bradley, and Kenneth J. Zucker, "Gender Identity Disorder." *Journal of the American Academy of Child Adolescent Psychiatry* 36.7 (1997): 872-80.

[105] Di Ceglie, "Gender Identity Disorder in Young People," 458.

[106] Bartlett, et al. "Is Gender Identity Disorder in Children a Mental Disorder?" 753.

one or more personality disorders, and 71% had currently, or at some time in their life, experienced Axis I disorders (e.g., depression, schizophrenia, social phobia).[107]

Hepp also noted that there are some authors who consider "Gender Dysphoria" as a result of an "underlying psychiatric comorbidity," while others consider the psychiatric comorbidities to be resulting from "persistent "Gender Dysphoria" and the concomitant psychosocial distress."

In her PhD Thesis, Wallien[108] found that "...*52% of the children diagnosed with GID had one or more diagnoses other than GID.*" She carefully analyzed her data with respect to comorbidity, and her analysis led her to conclude that "...*[it] is difficult to ascertain the relationship between psychopathology and gender dysphoria. If co-morbid conditions represent distinct disorders, one wonders whether one condition increases the risk for another condition, or whether the conditions are caused by distinct or overlapping factors. One often proposed explanation for the relationship between co-morbid problems and gender dysphoria is that the co-morbid problems are only a consequence of the gender dysphoria. It has been suggested that the gender dysphoric children's gender atypical behavior gives them a deviant social position, resulting in poor peer relations and victimization by peers. It has been argued that it is their deviant social status and/or*

---

[107] U. Hepp, B. Kraemer, U. Schnyder, et al., "Psychiatric Comorbidity in Gender Identity Disorder." *Journal of Psychosomatic Research* 58 (2005): 259-61.

[108] Madeleine S. C. Wallien, *Gender dysphoric children: Causes, Social functioning and Consequences* [Unpublished doctoral dissertation] (Vrije Universiteit Amsterdam, 2008), 86.

victimization that results in co-morbid psychiatric condition, probably through a mechanism of minority stress. <u>Our findings, however, give no reason to assume that minority stress is present in all gender dysphoric children</u>. In our study on the social status of gender-referred children, we did not find that they were victimized at school. Furthermore, considering the fact that more than half of the gender dysphoric children had co-morbid conditions in our DISC study, we find it unlikely that this diversity of co-morbid problems was solely the result of psychosocial stress. Considering our data on anxiety, <u>we believe it is more likely that the general vulnerability that seems to be present in many gender dysphoric children may also cause the co-morbid problems</u>. [my emphases]"[109]

After a clinical review of comorbidity in 10 patients interviewed at their clinic, Levine and Solomon "*...found 90% of these diverse patients had at least one other significant form of psychopathology.*"[110]

On the other hand, Meyer-Bahlburg cautioned against extrapolating too far from co-morbidity data. "*One has to realize, of course, that even if GID is associated with increased risk of other psychopathology, its definition as a mental disorder should stand on its own feet and not rely on 'co-morbidity' (in itself a term that implies GID as 'morbidity').*"[111]

---

[109] Ibid., 190.

[110] Levine and Solomon, "Meanings and Political Implications of "Psychopathology," 40-57.

[111] Meyer-Bahlburg, "From Mental Disorder to Iatrogenic Hypogonadism," 461.

Dhejne et al.[112] found that transsexual individuals had four times the number of hospitalizations for psychiatric morbidity (other than gender identity disorder) than controls prior to "SRS."

The American Psychiatric Association, in DSM-5, stated that "[clinically] *referred children with gender dysphoria show elevated levels of emotional and behavioral problems—most commonly, anxiety, disruptive and impulse-control, and depressive disorders. Clinically referred adolescents with gender dysphoria appear to have comorbid mental disorders, with anxiety and depressive disorders being the most common. As in children, autism spectrum disorder is more prevalent in clinically referred adolescents with gender dysphoria than in the general population. Clinically referred adults with gender dysphoria may have coexisting mental health problems, most commonly anxiety and depressive disorders.*"[113]

More recently, Meybodi et al. (2014), found that 81% of 73 patients seeking "SRS" had co-existing personality disorders.[114] It should be noted that the researchers actually excluded patients with Axis-I disorders (e.g., schizophrenia, mood and psychotic disorders) to *"decrease the effect of Axis-I disorders on the diagnosis of personality disorders."* So, this work only speaks to co-morbidity of personality disorders. Multiple disorders were present in most patients with the average number being three personality disorders.

---

[112] Cecilia Dhejne, Paul Lichtenstein, et al., "Long-Term Follow-Up of Transsexual Persons Undergoing Sex Reassignment Surgery: Cohort Study in Sweden." *PLoS ONE* 6.2: e16885. doi:10.1371/journal.pone.0016885.

[113] APA, DSM-5, 451.

[114] Azadeh M. Meybodi, Ahmad Hajebi, and Atefeh G. Jolfaei, "The Frequency of Personality Disorders in Patients with Gender Identity Disorder." *Medical Journal of the Islamic Republic of Iran* 28.90 (2014): 1-6.

In a study of 47 adolescents in Finland who were seeking "SRS", Kaltiala-Heino et al.[115] found that *"68% (32/47) had had their first contact with psychiatric services due to other reasons than gender identity issues."* In addition, 75% of the adolescents were being treated for other psychiatric disorders when they first sought "SRS."

Van Schalkwyk et al.[116] noted that there has been "…[an] *increasing number of reports [that] describe gender-related concerns in individuals with autism spectrum disorder (ASD)."* They indicate that many authors have found ASD to be "…*more common in individuals with a broad range of gender-related concerns…"*

It should be noted that although the studies all show significant psychiatric co-morbidities, Colizzi et al.[117] report that four studies have shown no co-morbidities. The main question is whether the subjects of these other studies were being treated with hormone therapy when the study was done. For example, the research Colizzi performed investigated gender dysphoric patients with Dissociative Identity Disorder (DID). Patients with DID can experience *"sexually oriented changes in alter-personalities."* They found the prevalence of dissociative disorder co-morbidities with "Gender Dysphoria" was

---

[115] Riittakerttu Kaltiala-Heino, Maria Sumia, et al., "Two years of gender identity service for minors: overrepresentation of natal girls with severe problems in adolescent development." *Child and Adolescent Psychiatry and Mental Health* (2015) 9:9 DOI 10.1186/s13034-015-0042-y.

[116] Gerrit I. Van Schalkwyk, Katherine Klingensmith, and Fred R. Volkmar, "Gender Identity and Autism Spectrum Disorders." *Yale Journal of Biology and Medicine* 88 (2015): 81-83.

[117] Marco Colizzi, Rosalia Costa, and Orlando Todarello, "Dissociative Symptoms in Individuals with Gender Dysphoria: Is the Elevated Prevalence Real?" *Psychiatry Research* 226.1 (March 30, 2015): 173-80.

more than twice that in the general population (29.6% vs 12.2%), and the existence of at least one major depressive episode in the subjects' lifetime was 45.8%. They also found that after treatment with hormone therapy, the co-morbidities were greatly reduced.

Kozlowska et al.[118] (2021) observed nearly 90% of child and adolescent patients in their study had co-morbid psychiatric diagnoses.

Janssen et al.[119] as cited in Sumia and Kaltiala[120] (2021) found that children with Autism Spectrum Disorder were almost 8 times more likely to express issues with their gender. Sumai and Kaltiala's research showed that "*All adolescents with gender dysphoria have more autism spectrum disorder than in the general population,*" and they had "*high percentages of psychiatric co-morbidities.*" They also showed that patients with "Gender Dysphoria" and Autism Spectrum Disorder had almost twice the risk (74% vs 49%, p=0.05) of "*self-harm/suicidality*" than adolescents with GD but no ASD.

Fisher et al.[121] note that "*the literature indicates a significant co-morbidity between schizophrenia and gender dysphoria.*" They present

---

[118] Kasia Kozlowska1, Catherine Chudleigh, et al., "Attachment Patterns in Children and Adolescents With Gender Dysphoria," *Frontiers in Psychology* 11 (January 2021): 1-21.

[119] Aron Janssen, Howard Huang, and Christina Duncan, "Gender variance among youth with autism spectrum disorders: A retrospective chart review." *Transgender Health* 1.1, (2016): 63-68.

[120] Maria Sumia and Riittakerttu Kaltiala, "Co-Occurring Gender Dysphoria and Autism Spectrum Disorder In Adolescence," *Psychiatria Fennica* 52 (2021): 104-114.

[121] Kristy A. Fisher, Samantha Scemla, et al., "Gender Dysphoria Versus Acute Psychosis: Can One Properly Diagnose Gender Dysphoria Solely During Acute Psychosis?" *HCA Healthcare Journal of Medicine* 3.3 (2022): 167-173.

a case study of a patient with *"gender identity variations coinciding solely with psychotic episodes during schizoaffective disorder, bipolar type."* In other words, the 35-year-old male patient experienced "Gender Dysphoria" **only** when he was also experiencing *"psychotic breaks of schizoaffective disorder, bipolar type."* The patient was treated with Risperidone (a commonly prescribed medicine for schizophrenia and bipolar disorder) and valproic acid (which is also used for bipolar disorder). In addition, he was treated with individual and group therapy. Within 8 days, the patient desisted[122] from his "Gender Dysphoria" and was discharged to his home.

Finally, the HHS report noted that there was a *"high rate (relative to the general population)"* of numerous co-morbidities, and *"75% of patients presenting to [Pediatric Gender Medicine] clinics in the mid-2010s had severe mental health problems that appeared to have pre-dated the emergence of GD."*[123]

While co-morbidities by themselves do not prove that "Gender Dysphoria" is a mental disorder, taken in aggregate with all of the other indicators, it is strongly suggestive of that fact.

<u>Argument from Similarity to Other Known Mental Disorders</u>

Interestingly, the co-morbidities presented from the literature above are similar to those present with many other true disorders. For example, from DSM-5 one can see:

---

[122] Desistance refers to an end to the feeling of being in the wrong body or an end to the desire of a patient to live as a member of the opposite sex.

[123] HHS, "Treatment for Pediatric Gender Dysphoria," 66-67.

- *"Individuals with <u>OCD</u> often have other psychopathology. Many adults with the disorder have a lifetime diagnosis of an anxiety disorder (76%; e.g., panic disorder, social anxiety disorder, generalized anxiety disorder, specific phobia) or a depressive or bipolar disorder (63% for any depressive or bipolar disorder, with the most common being major depressive disorder [41%])."* (pg. 242)

- *"Individuals with <u>Body Dysmorphic Disorder</u> often have "...major depressive disorder [which is] the most common comorbid disorder, with onset usually after that of body dysmorphic disorder. Comorbid social anxiety disorder (social phobia), OCD, and substance-related disorders are also common."* (pg. 247)

- *"Approximately 75% of individuals with <u>hoarding disorder</u> have a comorbid mood or anxiety disorder. The most common comorbid conditions are major depressive disorder (up to 50% of cases), social anxiety disorder (social phobia), and generalized anxiety disorder. Approximately 20% of individuals with hoarding disorder also have symptoms that meet diagnostic criteria for OCD."* (pg. 251)[124]

Note that all of these examples have major depressive disorders as co-morbidities. Similarly, Grant and Phillips studied women with anorexia who also had Body Dysmorphic Disorder (BDD) and found that *"shame and embarrassment"* contributed to underdiag-

---

[124] APA, DSM-5, 451.

nosis of BDD.[125] This "shame" must be from within, because nobody else knows that the women believe their bodies are fat. They don't have others shunning them because of the way they look. In fact, it is quite reasonable to assume that someone with a psychiatric disorder may be well-aware that there is something wrong or that they are different than others, even if they do not understand that they have a disorder. That could be the source of their depression. Similarly, if someone believes in their heart that they are trapped in the body of the wrong sex, and if people in positions of trust, such as psychiatric professionals, are affirming that, is it easy to imagine a straight-line extrapolation to symptoms of depression.

Some have said that the psychological co-morbidities associated with GID or "Gender Dysphoria" diagnoses are obviously the result of societal rejection. While that statement may sound reasonable, it defies the known patterns of mental disorders, which often present with multiple co-morbidities.

In fact, others have said that the co-morbidities are a sign that persons with GID are mentally ill to start and the GID is a symptom of the illness. For example, Meyer-Bahlburg acknowledged that "bi-directional causation cannot be ruled out."[126] However, McHugh cites a study by Meyer who followed up on adults who had received "SRS", and that study demonstrated that those adults "...*had much*

---

[125] Jon E. Grant, and Katharine A Phillips. "Is Anorexia Nervosa A Subtype Of Body Dysmorphic Disorder? Probably Not, But Read On?" *Harvard Review of Psychiatry* 12.2 (2004): 123-26.

[126] Meyer-Bahlburg, "From Mental Disorder to Iatrogenic Hypogonadism," 461.

the same problems with relationships, work and emotions as before."[127] This appears to indicate that the co-morbidities are evidence of a more general mental disorder.

Argument from Suicidality

Fitzgibbons, et al. (2009)[128] state that <u>seriously considering suicide is generally considered a symptom of mental illness</u>. It has been reported in the literature that the prevalence of suicide in the LGBT community, and especially in patients with "Gender Dysphoria," is higher than the general population.[129] Among the risk factors for suicide given by the American Association of Suicidology is *"interpersonal conflict in regard to sexual identity."*

Kenagy studied 182 transgendered people in the Philadelphia and Delaware Valley Regions and found that 30.1% of individuals had attempted suicide in the past.[130] In the study by Colizzi et al. the incidence of suicide attempts in those patients with "Gender Dysphoria" was 21.2%. According to the National Violent Death Report-

---

[127] Paul R. McHugh, "Surgical Sex: Why We Stopped Doing Sex Change Operations," *First Things* 11 (2004): 34-38.

[128] Richard P. Fitzgibbons, Philip M. Sutton, and Dale O'Leary, "The Psychopathology of "Sex Reassignment" Surgery - Assessing Its Medical, Psychological, and Ethical Appropriateness," *The National Catholic Bioethics Center* (Spring 2009): 97-125.

[129] American Association of Suicidology, *"Suicidal Behavior Among LGBT Youth Fact Sheet,"* https://suicidology.org/.

[130] Gretchen P. Kenagy, "Transgender Health: Findings from Two Needs Assessment Studies in Philadelphia." *Health & Social Work* 30.1 (2005): 19-26.

ing System, the rate of suicide attempts in the general population, for those who died by suicide was 20.6%.[131] Of those, 45.6% had a diagnosed mental disorder, and 74.6% of those had a diagnosis of depression or dysthymia (chronic, typically less severe, depression).

The rate for lifetime suicide attempts in the general population is 2.7%, with a range between 0.5 and 5.0%.[132] [133] Therefore, if the Kenagy study is generalizable, and using the Colizzi study outcome, the rate of suicide attempts among those with "Gender Dysphoria" ranges from a factor of 7 to 10 times that in the general population (n.b., the reader is cautioned that the sample size was extremely limited).

Similarly, LGBT advocates often cite the rate of suicide in patients with "Gender Dysphoria" as if it is different from other mental diseases. However, the rate of attempting suicide is very similar to that for patients with other mental illnesses as seen in the following studies.

Nock et al. [134] and the American Association of Suicidology[135] state that 9 out of 10 people who die by suicide had a diagnosable

---

[131] Centers for Disease Control and Prevention. Surveillance for Violent Deaths — National Violent Death Reporting System, 16 States, 2008. *Morbidity and Mortality Weekly Report* 60.10 (August 26, 2011): 2-49.

[132] Ronald C. Kessler, Guilherme Borges, and Ellen E. Walters. "Prevalence of and Risk Factors for Lifetime Suicide Attempts in the National Comorbidity Survey." *Archives of General Psychiatry* 56 (1999): 617-26.

[133] Matthew K. Nock, Guilherme Borges, et al., "Suicide and Suicidal Behavior." *Epidemiologic Reviews* 30.1 (2008): 133-54.

[134] Ibid., 133.

[135] American Association of Suicidology, "Know the Warning Signs Fact Sheet," https://suicidology.org/.

mental disorder. Among the risk factors cited are Major Axis I Psychiatric Disorders including "Body Dysmorphic Disorder." When examining the similarities and differences of BDD and Anorexia Nervosa, Grant and Phillips found that patients "*...who had anorexia plus BDD had ... three times the rate of suicide attempts [compared to anorexia alone] (63% vs. 20%).*"[136] Toomey et al. found that the rate of suicide attempts in transgender adolescents ranged from 30% to 50% depending on their gender identities. [137]

With respect to suicidality, the HHS report relates that "[s]*uicidal ideation and behavior are independently associated with comorbidities common among children and adolescents diagnosed with gender dysphoria...*" [and] "*No independent association between gender dysphoria and suicidality has been found...*"[138]

Risk factors specific for the LGBT community include social isolation, parental condemnation, depression, anxiety, and substance abuse, among others. It is unclear whether the psychiatric disorders are causative or a result of being transgender. According to Kenagy, in more than half of the people, being transgender was the reason they attempted suicide.[139]

Finally, Kessler et al. examined odds ratios for suicide attempts as a function of DSM-IIIR disorders and found that mood disorder has an odds ratio of 12.9, major depression of 11.0, and manias of

---

[136] Grant et al., "Is Anorexia Nervosa A Subtype," 123.

[137] Toomey, R.B., Syvertsen, A.K., Shramko, M.: "Transgender Adolescent Suicide Behavior," *Pediatrics*, 142.4 (2018) DOI: https://doi.org/10.1542/peds.2017- 4218.

[138] HHS, "Treatment for Pediatric Gender Dysphoria," 16.

[139] Kenagy, "Transgender Health," 19.

29.7.[140] Similarly, Brown et al. found that patients with major depressive disorders had an odds ratio of 9.59.[141] Therefore, as seen in Figure 1 (next page), the suicide rate for patients with "Gender Dysphoria" is similar to that of patients with mental disorders in general.

Argument from Ineffectiveness of "SRS"

Even with "treatments," it is clear that many individuals remain troubled, many continue to have significant psychiatric issues, and many regret their transitions. While the popular media does not acknowledge these, scientific literature does show evidence of this.

McHugh, a professor of psychiatry at Johns Hopkins University, recounted the rationale for the end to the practice of "SRS" at Johns Hopkins Hospital, where he was psychiatrist-in-chief.[142] He described a follow-up study of adults who had received sex-change operations wherein it was determined that "...*they were little changed in their psychological condition. They had much the same problems with relationships, work, and emotions as before. The hope that they would emerge now from their emotional difficulties to flourish psychologically had not been fulfilled.*"

A study by Reiner and Gearhart was included as a part of the Johns Hopkins reevaluation of the appropriateness of "SRS." Reiner and Gearhart evaluated the sexual integration of 16 children who

---

[140] Kessler et al., "Prevalence of and Risk Factors," 617.

[141] Gregory K. Brown, Aaron T. Beck, et al., "Risk Factors for Suicide in Psychiatric Outpatients: A 20-year Prospective Study." *Journal of Consulting and Clinical Psychology* 68.3 (2000): 371-77.

[142] McHugh, "Surgical Sex," 34.

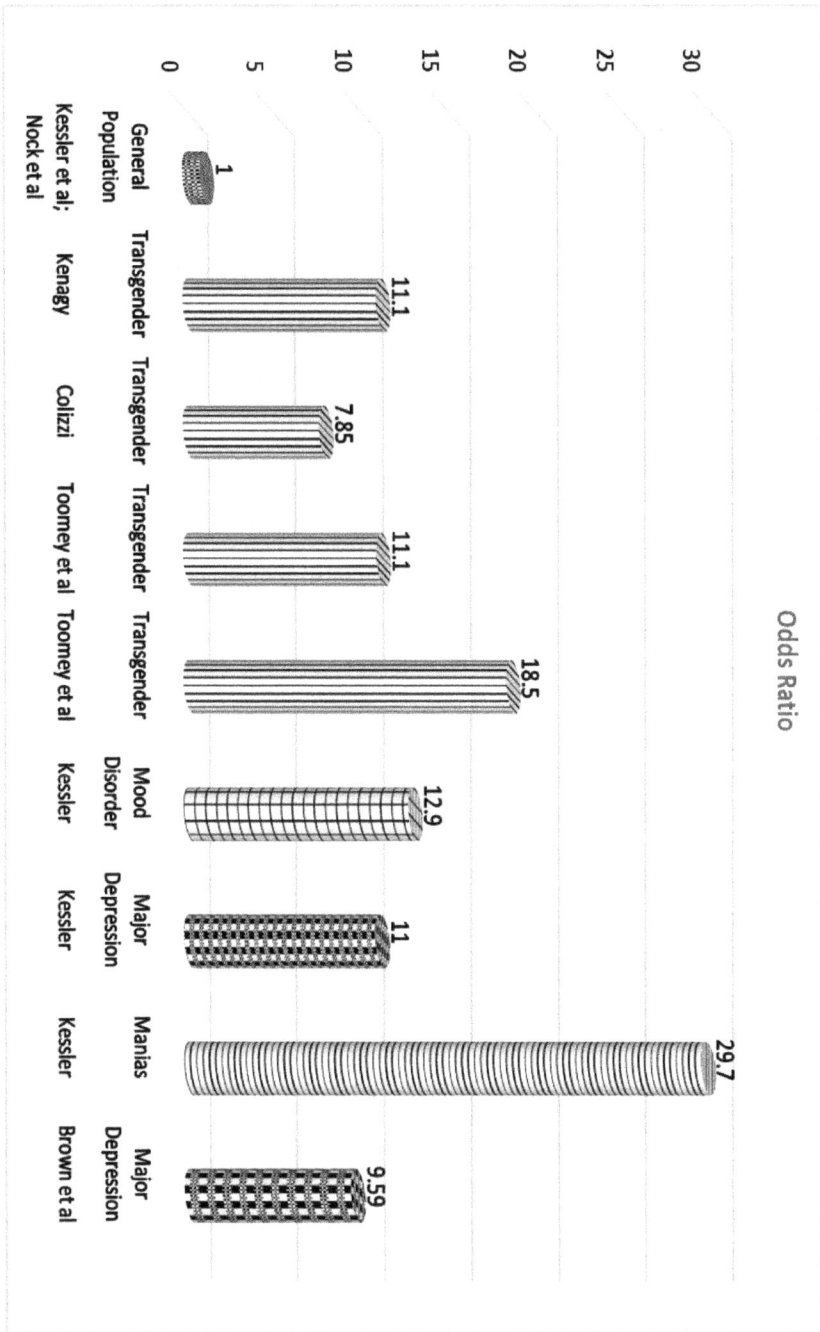

*Figure 1: Comparison of Odds Ratios for Suicide in General Population
(reference ratio), Transgender Population, and Population of Other Disorders*

were genetically male at birth, but who had a severe birth defect called cloacal exstrophy.[143] Because the condition results in severe genital deformities which are not typically surgically repairable, many of these children have "SRS" to make them resemble females. Their parents are then told to raise them as girls. Two of the sets of parents in this study refused the surgery and raised their children as males. Fourteen sets of parents had the surgery performed on their sons and raised them as girls. In their follow-up study, which was 5 to 16 years later, Reiner and Gearhart found that 8 of the 14 had declared themselves to be males and the 2 raised as males remained male. Of the remaining six children, five were living as females, and one was unclear of his or her sex. According to McHugh, then, from this study, Reiner concluded that *"the sexual identity followed the genetic constitution."*

Of even more concern is the study done by Dhejne et al.[144] They found that <u>postoperative</u> transexuals had 3 times the risk of psychiatric hospitalization, almost 5 times the risk of attempted suicide, and were over 19 times as likely to die by suicide when compared to control groups.

It's worth drilling into the study by Dhejne et al. a bit more. They found *"...substantially higher rates of overall mortality, death from cardiovascular disease and suicide, suicide attempts, and psychiatric*

---

[143] William G. Reiner and John P. Gearhart, "Discordant Sexual Identity in Some Genetic Males with Cloacal Exstrophy Assigned to Female Sex at Birth," *New England Journal of Medicine* 350.4 (January 22, 2004): 333–341.

[144] Dhejne, et al., "Long-Term Follow-Up," e16885.

hospitalizations in sex-reassigned transsexual individuals compared to a healthy control population."

They performed a nationwide, population-based, long-term follow-up of "sex-reassigned" transsexual persons and compared their cohort with randomly selected population controls matched for age and gender. *"The most striking result was the high mortality rate in both male-to-females and female-to males, compared to the general population. This contrasts with previous reports... that did not find an increased mortality rate after sex reassignment, or only noted an increased risk in certain subgroups."* They noted that there might be a built-in bias in previous clinical studies because *"people who regard their sex reassignment as a failure are more likely to be lost to follow-up."*

They also found that the risk of malignancies was increased by a factor of two (with *"borderline significance"*) and suggested that this was associated with the prolonged hormonal treatments that make up typical treatment plans. The malignancies noted in their study were lung cancer (N=3), tongue cancer (N=1), pharyngeal cancer (N=1), pancreatic cancer (N=1), hepatic cancer (N=1), and unknown origin (N=1).

Anecdotal reports of regret by people who had surgically transitioned are numerous such as one by Heyer, who said, *"Eventually, I gathered the courage to admit that the surgery had fixed nothing-it only masked and exacerbated deeper psychological problems."*[145]

---

[145] Walt Heyer, ""Sex Change" Surgery: What Bruce Jenner, Diane Sawyer, and You Should Know," *Public Discourse*, https://www.thepublicdiscourse.com/2015/04/14905/.

Similarly, according to Mayer and McHugh *"The scientific evidence [that they] summarized suggests we take a skeptical view toward the claim that sex-reassignment procedures provide the hoped-for benefits or resolve the underlying issues that contribute to the elevated mental health risks among the transgender population."*[146]

This view was further supported by two studies published in 2024. Straub et al., from U Texas Medical Branch in Galveston, compared suicide risk in patients who had "SRS" with several control groups.[147] They found that suicide risk in the population who had "SRS" was 12 times higher than the control group who had not experienced "SRS." Unfortunately, it was not clear whether any of the control groups were people with Gender Dysphoria who were not seeking "SRS." Nevertheless, the risk is right in line with the risk of suicide from other mental disorders mentioned in the previous section, showing that **"SRS" does not alleviate the suffering of patients with "Gender Dysphoria."**

Similarly, Ruuska et al. studied a nationally representative sample of individuals who entered nationally centralized gender identity clinics in Finland.[148] Those individuals were compared with matched population controls over a three-decade long follow-up period. The

---

[146] Mayer and McHugh, "Sexuality and Gender," 10.

[147] Straub, J.J., Paul, K.K., Bothwell, L.G., Deshazo, S.J., Golovko, G., Miller, M.S., Jehle, D.V. "Risk of Suicide and Self-Harm Following Gender-Affirmation Surgery." *Cureus* 16.4 (April 2, 2024): e57472. DOI 10.77559/cureus.57472.

[148] Sami-Matti Ruuska, Katinka Tuisku, Timo Holttinen, and Riittak-erttu Kaltiala, "All-cause and suicide mortalities among adolescents and young adults who contacted specialized gender identity services in Finland in 1996–2019: a register study." *British Medical Journal Mental Health* 27 (2024): 1–6. doi:10.1136/bmjment-2023-300940.

authors compared mortality from all causes and those from suicide in gender-referred adolescents as compared with matched controls. They observed that mortality from all causes was predicted by psychiatric treatment, with a higher risk associated with more occasions of treatment. They also found that patients experiencing "Gender Dysphoria" significant enough to ask for "SRS" did not have increased risk of death by suicide. Most importantly relative to the topic at hand, they found that **mortality from suicide did not differ between those who went through with "SRS" and those who did not**. They noted the following:

(1) *"[The main] predictor of mortality in this population is psychiatric morbidity"*

(2) *"...medical gender reassignment does not have an impact on suicide risk"*

(3) *"[this] does not support the claims that [Gender Reassignment Surgery] is necessary in order to prevent suicide"*

Previously, D'Angelo et al. noted, *"However, many of us, along with our colleagues, are seeing increasing numbers of detransitioners with adolescent-onset GD who regret not having received exploratory psychotherapy to help them understand their distress and the desire to transition before they underwent irreversible medical and surgical treatments."* [149]

---

[149] Roberto D'Angelo, Ema Syrulnik, et al., "One Size Does Not Fit All: In Support of Psychotherapy for Gender Dysphoria," *Archives of Sexual Behavior* 50 (2021): 7-16.

And Kaltiala observed that eight years after opening the first pediatric gender clinic in Finland, *"some previous patients started coming back to tell us they now regretted their transition. Some—called 'detransitioners'—wished to return to their birth sex."*[150] Fitzgibbons presents two famous individuals who underwent "SRS" only to regret those decisions.[151]

Most recently, the HHS report noted, *"the overall quality of evidence concerning the effects of any intervention on psychological outcomes, quality of life, regret, or long-term health, is very low."*[152] They further noted that while it's true that cross-sex hormone therapy and "SRS" alter the patient's appearance, *"[systematic reviews] have not found credible evidence that they lead to meaningful improvements in mental health."*[153]

Finally, with respect to the ineffectiveness of "SRS", the above-mentioned studies by McHugh, Mayer and McHugh, Dhejne et al., D'Angelo et al., Kaltiala-Heino et al., and Fitzgibbons, et al. have all shown that "SRS" is not the cure for "Gender Dysphoria." Patient suicides actually increase in some studies after "SRS." Many people who were transitioned as teens have come to regret their surgeries. A recent documentary highlights some of the experiences of 5 patients

---

[150] Riittakerttu Kaltiala, "Gender-Affirming Care Is Dangerous. I Know Because I Helped Pioneer It," The Free Press, https://www.thefp.com/p/ gender-affirming-care-dangerous-finland-doctor.

[151] Richard P. Fitzgibbons, "Transsexual attractions and sexual reassignment surgery: Risks and potential risks," The Linacre Quarterly Vol 82 No 4, 2015.

[152] HHS, "Treatment for Pediatric Gender Dysphoria," 13.

[153] HHS, "Treatment for Pediatric Gender Dysphoria," 76-77.

who had "SRS" and then regretted it only to detransition in the end.[154]

Similarly, Jennifer Lahl and Kallie Fell, in their book, "The Detransition Diaries," document the experiences of five women and two men who experienced "Gender Dysphoria" and had transitioned to varying degrees before realizing that it was a mistake.[155] While seven is a small sample size, the authors note that *"the detrains group on Reddit, at the time of this writing [©2024], has more than 48,000 members, up from 13,000 in June 2020."* If hormone therapy and "SRS" were effective, one would not expect to see such numbers.

Argument from the Deficiencies in the Development of the DSM and Standards in General

The HHS report examined the role of medical and mental health associations in the development of Standard of Care Guidelines.[156] They observed that these associations *"are not immune to institutional biases, including groupthink and the disproportionate influence of vocal, specialized subcommittees."*

Davies[157] described the process of the development of DSM-III. The process consisted of APA's Council of Research and Development initiating a Task Force and choosing a Chair. They chose

---

[154] https://nowaybackfilm.com/, 2023.

[155] Jennifer Lahl and Kallie Fell, *The Detransition Diaries*, (San Francisco: Ignatius Press, 2024), page 177.

[156] HHS, "Treatment for Pediatric Gender Dysphoria," 204.

[157] James Davies, "How Voting and Consensus Created the Diagnostic and Statistical Manual of Mental Disorders (DSM-III)," *Anthropology & Medicine* 24.1 (2017): 34-36.

Robert Spitzer who had a major role in developing DSM-II, and who had helped to declassify homosexuality as a mental disorder in 1973. Spitzer then was given free rein to choose members of the Task Force. The Task Force started out as 8 members and grew to 15 members to allow different perspectives to be considered. Of critical importance, however, was the fact that inclusion of individuals with **psychoanalytic expertise was intentionally kept to a minimum.**

In the development of DSM-III a consensus process was used to include disorders. Davies noted that "the word *'consensus' does not necessarily denote the consensus of the wider psychiatric or mental health community. While it was certainly true that wider consensus was tested and sought among psychiatrists (i.e. through questionnaires petitioning selected APA members for views on certain Task Force proposals), the consensus that really mattered was that reached by the Task Force itself, whose prime occupation was to be the final arbiter of any proposed change or inclusion."* As the HHS report authors note, "[c]*onsensus does not guarantee correctness—in fact, it can sometimes entrench error.*"[158]

As is the case with development of many scientific standards, a small group of interested parties is pulled together to constitute a committee. Often these committees consist of technical experts and interested parties, who may be non-technical or people with technical background in a related field, but not considered experts in the subject matter.

In my over 30 years of work on standards within the Society of Automotive Engineers (SAE), I chaired and participated in many

---

[158] HHS, "Treatment for Pediatric Gender Dysphoria," 25.

such committees. I have a lot of experience with committee members who had political agendas and those sent to prevent a standard from being implemented or at least slow down its progress. One standard on which I was the principal author took 25 years to develop, in part, because there was significant pushback from some members of the committee. This push back was in the form of political comments veiled as scientific comments which had to be addressed. When the standard was finally drafted, it was sent to a broader group for a vote. Often this would result in some comments that were reasonable and some that were irrelevant but had to be addressed, leading to the need for multiple versions and multiple votes, causing the process to drag on.

When they are finally approved, technical standards remain the work product of a relatively small number of people, who do not necessarily represent the views of the rest of the scientific community. In fact, even if a standard was sent to the entire membership list of SAE safety subcommittees, very few would have the time to actually give the standard a detailed review.

Evidently, according to Davies, the development of DSM was very similar in some respects.[159] However, in some very important respects it was different. The committee that developed DSM-III was selected by Robert Spitzer who had helped develop DSM-II. He played a *"decisive role in declassifying homosexuality as a mental disorder in 1973,"* and may have had an inherent bias against gender identity disease as a mental disorder. Spitzer himself was the sole judge of who would be on his committee. Davies further noted that

---

[159] Ibid.

committee decisions were made by consensus which did not include input from the broader psychiatric or mental health community.

The contribution of <u>social and political factors</u> in the description of "Gender Dysphoria" in the DSM was acknowledged by Beek et al.[160] The second author on Beek's paper was well-informed on this subject given that she was "*chair of the American Psychiatric Association's DSM-5 GID Subworkgroup of the Workgroup on Sexual and GIDs.*"

The most troublesome concern regarding the development comes from a quote, attributed by Davies, to Robert Spitzer himself. "*Indeed, as Spitzer stated in interview: 'Our team was certainly not typical of the psychiatry community, and that was one of the major arguments against DSM III: **it allowed a small group with a particular viewpoint to take over psychiatry and change it in a fundamental way**'. When asking Spitzer what he made of that criticism, he responded: 'What did I think of that charge? - **Well, it was absolutely true. It was a revolution, that's what it was. We took over because we had the power'.*"[161]

According to Davies, "*...the construction of DSM-IV and indeed DSM-5 did not differ in any fundamental way from the basic procedures DSM-III followed... committee consensus remained at the core of all decision-making.*"[162] And, according to Davies, "*...the DSM cumulative project... accumulated over consecutive editions has been the **product of processes and decisions prone to bias and error...**"*

---

[160] Beek, et al., "Gender incongruence, 5.
[161] Davies, "How Voting and Consensus Created, 34.
[162] Ibid.

Again, the HHS report authors note the expectations of the National Academy of Medicine for the development of "clinical practice guidelines."[163] Among those expectations is a systematic review of the studies in the literature, coupled with experts from multiple fields that bear on the subject matter, and a minimization of conflicts of interest and biases.

In the end, if the decision to remove the classification of Gender Identity Disorder as a mental disorder was made by a small committee, Davies suggests it may not represent the opinion of the broader mental health community. Those who are practicing in the field may not have been presented with an analysis like the present one, and like those in many scientific fields may be accepting the opinion of a committee with a political agenda and personal biases. In the current environment, "[w]*hen medical societies update their treatment guidelines and position statements, experts who question the evidence supporting PMT are excluded from guideline development committees.*"[164]

As the HHS report points out, "*the American Psychiatric Association's (APA) 'Guideline for Gender Affirming Psychiatric Care (GAPC)' has faced internal criticism for failing to acknowledge the scientific debate and the policy shifts occurring internationally.*"[165]

Meyer-Bahlburg considered the fact that the mechanisms of "Gender Dysphoria" are unknown or not fully understood to mean that we can't call it a mental disorder.[166] Cancer is proof that one

---

[163] HHS, "Treatment for Pediatric Gender Dysphoria," 133-134.

[164] HHS, "Treatment for Pediatric Gender Dysphoria," 209-210.

[165] HHS, "Treatment for Pediatric Gender Dysphoria," 206.

[166] Meyer-Bahlburg, "From Mental Disorder to Iatrogenic Hypogonadism," 461.

doesn't need to know the cause of something to know that it is pathological. The same lack of knowledge of the etiology can be said of Body Integrity Disorder or many other mental disorders, but that has not removed them from consideration as disorders. Why is "Gender Dysphoria" treated differently? I would argue that it is treated differently because of society's idolization of all things sexual and because of the pressure from advocacy groups and politicians.

Even if a biological cause is found, that does not diminish the fact that "Gender Dysphoria" is a mental disorder. Much of clinical depression is believed to be biochemical in origin.[167] That doesn't mean it's not a mental disorder. On the plus side, however, because there are clues to its origins, pharmaceutical agents have been developed to bring the mind some relief. If "Gender Dysphoria" is not considered a mental disorder, there will never be research to see if a pharmaceutical agent can ease or eliminate the symptoms.

It seems fitting to end this section with a quote from psychiatrist, Dr. Miriam Grossman[168] who stated, "*Once I understood who the founders [of modern American sexual education] were, I knew how we reached today's madness. It came from disturbed individuals with dangerous ideas – radical activists who wanted to create a society that would not only accept their pathology, but celebrate it!*"

---

[167]   https://www.mayoclinic.org/diseases-conditions/depression/symptoms-causes/syc-20356007.

[168] Miriam Grossman, "A Brief History of Sex Ed: How We Reached Today's Madness." *Public Discourse*, https://www.thepublicdiscourse.com/2013/07/10408/.

Conclusions to Part One

When the people in the general public hear the term "Gender Dysphoria," they think it means someone who is confused about their "gender." A male who thinks he is really a female or a female who thinks she is really a male. They have been told by the APA, and subsequently by all the major medical establishments, that "Gender Dysphoria" is not a mental disorder. What they have not been told, is that the APA "Working Group on Sexual and Gender Identity Disorders," has manipulated the language in the DSM to intentionally mislead the public. Since most people have not examined the scientific literature on the subject, they have no way of knowing this fact. The APA states[169] *"the presence of gender variance is not the pathology but dysphoria is from the distress caused by the body and mind not aligning and/or social marginalization of gender-variant people."* This is a classic lie of misdirection. Their position appears to be that the patient is not suffering from a delusion, but that since scientific biologically demonstrable <u>facts differ from the patient's feelings</u>, <u>it must be the facts that are wrong</u>.

In their fact sheet with general information on "Gender Dysphoria," the APA notes that *"DSM-5 aims to avoid stigma…"*[170] Similarly, literature on the APA website explains the rationale for changes to

---

[169] Gender Dysphoria Diagnosis, https://www.psychiatry.org/psychiatrists/diverstiy/education/transgender-and-gender-nonconforming-patients/gender-dysphoria-diagnosis.

[170] https://www.psychiatry.org/file%20library/psychiatrists/practice/dsm/apa_dsm-5-gender-dysphoria.pdf.

DSM-5TR's terminology.[171] Changing terms, for example, from *"cross-sex medical procedure"* to *"gender-affirming medical procedure,"* was done to use *"culturally-sensitive and less stigmatizing language."* That terminology may seem compassionate, but it is a false compassion and is misguided and misleading at best. Objectively speaking, if a patient with Anorexia, Bipolar Disorder, or Body Dysmorphic Disorder was offended by their diagnosis, would a psychiatric professional change the diagnosis?

In this author's view, there is a preponderance of clear and convincing evidence, to come to the conclusion that **the gender variance associated with "Gender Dysphoria" <u>DOES</u>** constitute a mental disorder, in and of itself. Therefore, since **gender identity variance IS a mental disorder** whether or not the patient reports associated distress, **"Gender Identity Disorder"** should be added back into the DSM. As shown, the evidence for this statement includes significant deviation from the mathematical norm of the population, common understanding of biology, tendency away from species survival, significant psychiatric co-morbidities that follow the same pattern as other recognized disorders, similarity to other known mental disorders, suicide rates similar to other mental disorders, and ineffectiveness of "SRS" at resolving associated psychiatric conditions.

The APA essentially proves the point that gender variance <u>IS a mental disorder</u> in their own DSM. From DSM-5[172], the **<u>definition of a "mental disorder"</u>** is:

---

[171]   https://www.psychiatry.org/getmedia/a5bef7b8-d401-4fc2-bac5-21a4d788fdb6/APA-DSM5TR-GenderDysphoria.pdf.

[172] APA, DSM-5, pp. 20-21; DSM-5-TR, pp. 14-15.

*"A mental disorder is a syndrome characterized by clinically significant disturbance in an individual's cognition, emotion regulation, or behavior that reflects a dysfunction in the psychological, biological, or developmental processes underlying mental functioning. **Mental disorders are usually associated with significant distress** or disability in social, occupational, or other important activities.*

Each mental disorder in the DSM contains a list of the diagnostic criteria for the disorder:

*"...**a generic diagnostic criterion requiring distress or disability has been used to establish disorder thresholds**, usually worded "the disturbance causes clinically significant distress or impairment in social, occupational, or other important areas of functioning."*

What these two statements mean is that a mental disorder is characterized by a person's disordered thought processes or behavior that lead to distress. There is a subtle, but critical difference in the diagnostic criteria for "Gender Dysphoria."

According to DSM-5-TR[173], the Diagnostic Criteria for "Gender Dysphoria" in both children and adults, require **two** main conditions:

---

[173] APA, DSM-5-TR, pp. 513-514.

"A. A marked <u>**incongruence between one's experienced/ex-**</u><u>**pressed gender and assigned gender**</u>, *of at least 6 months' du-ration, as manifested by...*"

AND

"B. *The condition is* <u>**associated with clinically significant dis-**</u><u>**tress**</u> *or impairment in social, school, or other important ar-eas of functioning.*"

That is, the "distress" had been separated from the main criteria as if it is not related to the disordered thought processes or behavior. As noted earlier, from DSM-5, ""*Gender Dysphoria refers to* <u>**the dis-**</u><u>**tress**</u> *that may accompany the incongruence between one's experi-enced or expressed gender and one's assigned gender* [my empha-sis]."[174] Then, the DSM states that it is the state of distress, called "dysphoria," that is the mental disorder, not the disordered thoughts or behavior.

The APA Working Group on "Sexual and Gender Identity Disor-ders" appears determined to have it both ways. This is in fact what one of its members said, when they admitted that the "...*main di-lemma in the DMS-5 was to reduce stigma while securing access to care for those individuals who need it.*"[175] On the one hand, claiming that "gender variance" is <u>not</u> a "Mental Disorder," and on the other hand, stating that "Gender Dysphoria" is a mental disorder.

Again, in order to be diagnosed with "Gender Dysphoria" the patient's condition must be "**associated with clinically significant**

---

[174] APA, DSM-5, 451.
[175] Beek, et al., "Gender incongruence, 5.

distress or impairment in social, occupational or other important areas of functioning," but the underlying condition of gender variance, or confusion in gender identity, is <u>not</u> considered a mental disorder. According to DSM-5 (pg. 21), <u>distress is the threshold criterion for a clinically significant "mental disorder."</u>[176] [177] But that criterion is contained within the diagnostic criteria of other mental disorders, such as Body Dysmorphic Disorder.[178] "Distress" is intentionally called out separately for "Gender Dysphoria."

This fraud has been perpetuated on the unsuspecting and well-meaning citizens of the world who have no means of reading all the literature and forming their own opinions. What Beek et al. state, is worth repeating in full:

> "In DSM-5, a new specifier was added to include individuals who have undergone at least one somatic intervention or treatment that affirms their experienced gender (e.g. cross-sex hormone treatment)... This implies that individuals who were once diagnosed with gender dysphoria can 'lose' the diagnosis. Yet for those who need a diagnosis for access to care (e.g. cross-sex hormone treatment) this is still possible with this specifier..."[179]

The translation of this paragraph is something like this: 'Yes, it's a mental disorder, when I want insurance companies (viz., other

---

[176] APA, DSM-5, 21.

[177] Jack Drescher, "Controversies in Gender Diagnoses," LGBT Health 1.1 (2013): 1-5.

[178] APA, DSM-5, 242.

[179] Beek, et al., "Gender incongruence, 5.

people) to pay the bills for 'treatment,' but no it's not a mental disorder once the treatment is done or for those who choose not to go on to chemical or surgical treatment." This is the same position as the ICD-11 Working Group proposing changes to the ICD-10 in 2012.[180]

Political considerations and ideologies, combined with the deficiencies of standards development processes, especially in the development of the DSM, have led to the rejection of gender variance, or gender identity confusion, as a mental disorder. Because the DSM is considered the ground truth for psychiatric and psychological matters, this falsehood has been forced on society as a whole by unsuspecting professional organizations such as the AMA and AAP, whose members have relied on the APA to provide scientifically reliable information. This is not unusual as noted in the HHS report because *"in managing unusual or complex conditions, primary care providers and generalist clinicians often rely on the expertise of specialists to inform their clinical decisions."*[181] However, in the face of so much debate in the scientific community, those organizations have a responsibility to perform critical reviews of the literature to form their own opinions.

Given the way standards are developed, it is likely that the broader mental health community had no input on the declassification of Gender Identity Disorder by a small group with a political agenda. To use the words of Levine and Solomon, *"promotion of civil rights for the transgendered* [appear to have obscured] *professional*

---

[180] Jack Drescher, et al., "Minding the body," 568.

[181] HHS, "Treatment for Pediatric Gender Dysphoria," 207.

perceptions of psychopathology."[182] However, it is clear to an objective outside scientific observer that gender variance/confusion specifically, and "Gender Dysphoria" as a whole, is a mental disorder. The implication of this is that Gender Identity Disorder should be added back into the DSM and considered a mental disorder by the APA, AMA, AAP, and WHO.

While the term "mental disorder" may be perceived as having negative connotations associated with it in mainstream society, NOT calling gender variance or "Gender Dysphoria" (as the public knows it) a mental disorder does not help patients come to grips with the reality of the situation. Not calling "Gender Dysphoria" a mental disorder, may sound compassionate, but it is false compassion. Using an analogy from physical medicine, if I should tell a patient that they have a physical cellular condition rather than saying they have cancer, because of the trauma associated with that diagnosis, I have not done the patient any great service. Nor will that change the fact that they are physically ill and in need of physical and or pharmaceutical help. By not stating the truth to them, they may avoid the treatments that they need to stay alive. Similarly, by "affirming" "Gender Dysphoria" in patients, psychologists are keeping them from seeking the psychological counseling and treatment that may truly help them. Instead, they become more determined to move into the dangerous world of potentially irreversible cross-sex hormone therapies and the world of certainly irreversible physical organ removal.

Numerous psychological conditions, including many of those which are often co-morbidities of "Gender Dysphoria," have

---

[182] Levine and Solomon, "Meanings and Political Implications of "Psychopathology," 40-57.

benefited from various forms of psychotherapy.[183] Not acknowledging the fact that the gender variance which leads to "Gender Dysphoria" is a mental disorder steers patients away from therapeutic approaches that may actually help them.

Reclassifying "Gender Dysphoria" as a mental disorder may also help to stop the exponential rise in cases among teens for whom this has become a cause célèbre. In the last five years, *"the number of young people claiming to be "trans" has more than doubled with no sign of slowing."* [184]

There is one matter on which this author agrees with the APA and ICD-11 working groups. There should be no *"discrimination against transgender individuals."*[185] No one with a mental disorder should be subjected to prejudice or inhumane treatment. People with "Gender Dysphoria" are real human beings who are suffering. They should be loved, and accompanied by others, not ridiculed or tormented. Such behaviors themselves are immoral.

However, not being truthful about a condition, whether for political reasons, or to prevent stigmatization, is also immoral. The psychiatric, psychological, and medical professions should accept the fact that this condition is a mental disorder and make this known to government policy makers.

Asking society as a whole to participate in a mental disorder by using the "correct pronouns," allowing genetic men into women's restrooms and changing rooms, allowing men to participate in

---

[183] HHS, "Treatment for Pediatric Gender Dysphoria," 251-252, 257-258.

[184] Lahl and Fell, The Detransition Diaries, 175.

[185] Drescher, "Controversies," 1.

women's sports, etc. is lunacy and deprives the majority of society of their rights. Is it ethical to put the majority at risk to enable a minority to have their way? Societies that value freedom understand that protecting the inalienable rights of minorities is a laudable objective. But so is protecting the rights of the majority. Allowing people with a mental disorder to use cross-sex bathrooms, for example, has great potential for harm of those in society who are in the majority as news reports have shown.[186]

The recent Olympics boxing match that included two male-to-female transexuals is a case in point.[187] The natal women who were paired against them had no chance. Italian boxer Angela Carini, who faced one of the men, had previously won a medal at the 2019 AIBA Women's World Boxing Championships. After facing the male in the Olympics, she stated that she had never been hit so hard in her life and quit the match in 46 seconds after years of training. This should come as no surprise. It's well documented that human males have *"approximately 60% more muscle mass and nearly 90% more overall strength"* than females.[188]

---

[186] Caroline Downey, "Judge Rules Loudoun County Teen Sexually Assaulted Female Student in Girls' Bathroom," *Yahoo* (October 26, 2021) https://www.yahoo.com/news/judge-rules-loudoun-county-teen-131413442.html.

[187] Ingrid Jacques, "Olympic boxers deserve compassion. But questions of fairness shouldn't be brushed aside." *USA Today* (August 6, 2024) https://www.usatoday.com/story/opinion/columnist/2024/08/06/olympic-boxer-controversy-fairness-sports-title-ix/74679486007/.

[188] Cara Buskmiller and Paul Hruz, "A Biological Understanding of Man and Woman," 59-97.

"Gender Dysphoria" clearly is real to the patients who experience it. Otherwise, who would be willing to risk losing loved ones by transitioning, or who would undergo painful life-altering surgeries? Patients are suffering. The key question is what should be done to help them? Males and females are a composite of a spectrum of behaviors. There are effeminate men, masculine women and everything in between. Being nurturing doesn't mean that a male is any less a man. Being tough doesn't mean that a female is any less a woman.

There has been a societal movement to normalize every kind of sexually deviant behavior and gender ideology is no different. Given that fact, a fitting end to this section is a quote from pediatrician, Dr. Michelle Cretella, "*Truth is the enemy of the sexual revolution. Reality itself must be suppressed for the full sexual agenda to be realized.*"[189]

Proposed Actions from Part One:

- The APA, AAP, AMA, and WHO should either bring the "Gender Identity Disorder" diagnosis back into the DSM or rename "Gender Dysphoria" with a name that reflects it as a mental disorder if either of the two diagnostic criteria are met.

  o The organization should unequivocally state this publicly.

---

[189] Life Site News, "LGBT activists slam 'the most important psychiatrist of the last half century' because he debunks transgender ideology", https://www.lifesitenews.com/news/lgbtactivists.

- Given that a small group determined the declassification of Gender Identity Disorder as a mental disorder, the broader APA community should hold a special meeting to debate the facts as presented here and issue a referendum to the community of practicing psychiatrists and psychologists who deal with individuals affected by it.

  o If the APA leadership refuses to do this, those who pay dues every year, should use the power of the purse and withhold their dues payments until the issue is resolved.
  o If that doesn't work the APA should be disbanded and a new organization created which considers all aspects of this issue from a scientific standpoint aside from political influences of lobbying and advocacy organizations.

- The APA, AAP, AMA, and WHO should make it clear that those affected with "Gender Dysphoria" are in need of psychological help (cross-hormone therapy and "SRS" are not appropriate treatments as will be discussed in Part Two).
- Once this unambiguous reclassification of "Gender Dysphoria" as a mental disorder is done, lawmakers around the world need to hear from these organizations to repeal laws that criminalize psychotherapy as a treatment for "Gender Dysphoria" and instead should mandate it.
- These same lawmakers should also enact laws that prohibit sex "reassignment" surgeries, especially on minors/ adolescents. Those in the medical community should refuse to

perform these procedures, especially when psychological treatments have not been sought first.

-   Governments should allocate resources to perform genuine scientific research on the causes and treatments; especially psychotherapeutic treatments and benign pharmaceutical treatments aimed at bringing the mind back to reality or at least reducing the distress associated with the disorder. These steps are far more likely to help the greatest number of individuals with "Gender Dysphoria" (see Part Two).

PART TWO

WHAT ARE ETHICAL TREATMENTS
FOR "GENDER DYSPHORIA"?

Abstract

Having established, in Part One, that "Gender Dysphoria" is a mental disorder, I explore ethical ways to manage it based on the same extensive review of the literature as in Part One. The special cases of children and adolescents are considered separately. In addition to discussing what constitutes ethical treatment, I also explore what must be considered unethical treatments such as puberty blocking drugs, cross-sex hormone therapy to initiate transitioning, and "gender-affirming surgery". A set of proposed actions is included to give suggestions for ways to actually help patients who genuinely suffer with this disorder.

Introduction

In Part One, I summarized the evidence leading to the conclusion that the gender variance associated with "Gender Dysphoria," and therefore, the whole construct of "Gender Dysphoria," is a mental disorder.[1] From that review, it is abundantly clear that the etiology

---

[1] In this part, I will continue to capitalize the term "Gender Dysphoria" and put it in quotation marks unless it is used in a direct quote. In that case, I will follow the style of the paper being cited.

79

of "Gender Dysphoria" is unknown. For example, is it a neuroanatomic disorder, a biochemical disorder, or is it a result of some other
unknown pathology?

According to many in the APA, and particularly in advocacy
groups, "gender-affirming" treatment is the only compassionate
treatment for "Gender Dysphoria." However, "gender-affirming"
treatment, which may begin with social affirmation, often leads to
medical interventions to alter the patient's body. This starts with a
regimen of cross-sex hormones and, for some patients, ultimately
leads to "gender-affirming surgery," also mistakenly labeled "sex reassignment surgery," in which a person's anatomy is surgically
changed to resemble that of the opposite sex.[2] During this surgery,
healthy tissues are excised from the patient's body and discarded. The
patient must then remain on cross-sex hormones for life. As will be
shown, in this author's view, calling these steps "treatment" is dis-
honest at best. The mechanism by which people become gender dysphoric is not known, but there is evidence that it can be resolved in
some cases by psychological counseling.

In a 2017 news article about "Gender Dysphoria," Dr. Paul
McHugh, University Distinguished Service Professor of Psychiatry
at the Johns Hopkins University School of Medicine stated something that should be obvious to any intelligent human being but has
eluded many of those in modern psychiatry. Namely that, "*A doctor
who prescribes treatment should understand the nature of the problem*

---

[2] In this part, I will continue to use the term 'sex "reassignment" surgery' with "reassignment" in quotes, or "SRS" also in quotes, unless it is
used in a direct quote. In that case, I will follow the style of the paper being
cited.

he is treating."[3] Yet, the fact that the etiology is unknown has not prevented dangerous "treatments" in the name of compassion. Nevertheless, as will be discussed, this is a false compassion fed by ideology and not by science.

Such was the case in the 1930s through 1950s when pre-frontal lobotomies were the rage in an attempt to "cure" all kinds of mental disorders. However, as Gostin reports, "*...the surgery was used predominantly for schizophrenia where there was little evidence of its positive effect. More importantly, there were potentially serious side effects which included intellectual and emotional impairment and personality change... prolonged incontinence, epilepsy and certain metabolic disorders.*"[4] Although limited psychosurgery is still performed today, it has a more established scientific basis with much better outcomes.

In this second part, I will review a number of studies that propose a reasonable etiology for "Gender Dysphoria," namely, that is a function of some traumatic event in the early years of a person's life. This hypothesis would indicate very different treatment regimens than those currently advocated by the APA, AMA, AAP, and WHO – so called "gender-affirming care."

---

[3] Life Site News, "LGBT activists slam 'the most important psychiatrist of the last half-century' because he debunks transgender ideology," May 15, 2017, https://www.lifesitenews.com/news/lgbt-activists-slam-the-most-important-psychiatrist-of-the-last-half-centur/.

[4] Larry O. Gostin, "Ethical considerations of psychosurgery: the unhappy legacy of the pre-frontal lobotomy," *Journal of Medical Ethics* 6 (1980): 149-154.

What is "treatment" for "Gender Dysphoria" if it is a mental disorder?

People with "Gender Dysphoria" are human beings who are truly suffering. Simple human compassion demands that the condition be appropriately acknowledged. It also demands reasonable attempts to address the condition and provide relief to the individuals so afflicted, based on scientific reason and not on political considerations.

In a book published in 1966, by Harry Benjamin, one of the fathers of the transgender movement, Benjamin wrote, "*Psychotherapy with the aim of curing transsexualism, so that the patient will accept himself as a man... is a useless undertaking __with present available methods__ [my emphasis]. The mind of the transsexual cannot be changed in its false gender orientation. All attempts to this effect have failed* (as cited in Lahl and Fell)."[5]

Similarly, the APA states:

> "*Support for people with gender dysphoria may include open-ended exploration of their feelings and experiences of gender identity and expression, without the therapist having any pre-defined gender identity or expression outcome defined as preferable to another.*
>
> *Psychological attempts to force a transgender person to be cisgender (sometimes referred to as gender identity conversion efforts*

---

[5] Harry Benjamin, *The Transsexual Phenomenon* (New York: The Julian Press, Inc., 1966), 91, quoted in Jennifer Lahl and Kallie Fell, *The Detransition Diaries*, (San Francisco: Ignatius Press, 2024), 26.

or so-called "gender identity conversion therapy") are considered unethical and have been linked to adverse mental health outcomes.

Support may also include affirmation in various domains. Social affirmation may include an individual adopting pronouns, names, and various aspects of gender expression that match their gender identity. Legal affirmation may involve changing name and gender markers on various forms of government identification. Medical affirmation may include pubertal suppression for adolescents with gender dysphoria and gender-affirming hormones like estrogen and testosterone for older adolescents and adults. Medical affirmation is not recommended for prepubertal children. Some adults (and less often adolescents) may undergo various aspects of surgical affirmation."[6]

Today, despite Benjamin's and the APA's claims, there IS evidence for the success of psychological treatments in cases of patients with "Gender Dysphoria." Real treatment for a mental disorder is treatment that helps the mind experience reality as it is. In the case of "Gender Dysphoria," that would mean helping the mind experience the reality of the body. In some cases that may mean pharmacological interventions, but in all cases, it should begin with psychological therapy.

Nicolosi, Byrd, and Potts[7] demonstrated that psychological therapy was effective in many patients with diverse sexual behaviors.

---

[6] APA, "What is Gender Dysphoria?" https://www.psychiatry.org/patients-families/gender-dysphoria/what-is-gender-dysphoria.

[7] Joseph Nicolosi, A. Dean Byrd, and Richard W. Potts. "Retrospective Self-Reports Of Changes In Homosexual Orientation: A Consumer Survey

Therefore, it's not unreasonable to expect that "Gender Dysphoria" will also respond when the correct treatment is found. This implies, however, that the causes must be determined, that someone is looking for them, and that patients will want to be helped.

Di Ceglie presents three case studies of individuals suffering from "Gender Dysphoria." [8] While not all of the cases desisted, all seemed to benefit from long term psychotherapy. Importantly, Di Ceglie noted that in some cases what he called "*Atypical Gender Identity Organization*" can develop in early childhood subsequent to some traumatic event. In some cases, he believes the individual may be amenable to change whereas in others it may not be. He also expressed a belief that the first step in management of gender identity disorder is "*therapeutic exploration*," and that "*[s]urgical intervention cannot be justified until adulthood.*"

Korte et al.[9] also showed that, in many cases, "Gender Dysphoria" was due to early traumas or childhood difficulties, and they resolved with psychological counseling. They noted that if "*...psychodynamically relevant conflicts and "transsexualogenic" factors that may be present [are] thoroughly analyzed and worked through in psychotherapy or family therapy... there is a real chance that the patient will, in the end, no longer desire a sex change.*"

Of Conversion Therapy Clients." *Psychological Reports* 86.3c (2000): 1071-088.

[8] Domenico Di Ceglie, "Gender Identity Disorder in Young People." *Advances in Psychiatric Treatment* 6 (2000): 458-66.

[9] Alexander Korte, David Goecker, et al., "Gender Identity Disorders in Childhood and Adolescence." *Deutsches Arzteblatte International* 105.48 (2008): 834-41.

Fitzgibbons et al. explain that many patients with "Gender Dysphoria" "...*have been victims of various forms of abuse or neglect and of peer or parental rejection. Basic emotional needs for secure attachment relationships to same-sex peers and to the same-sex parent have often not been met. Gender dysphoria is rarely their only diagnosable psychological disorder.*"[10]

Similarly, Fitzgibbons[11] noted "*Children who seek SRS should be evaluated for psychological conflicts but regularly are not.*" He also notes the success of his own clinic and others in helping children "*develop skills associated with children of their own biological sex*" and helping them to develop friendships.

Kaltiala-Heino et al. found that of the 47 adolescents seeking "SRS" in their study in Finland, "[seventy percent] *(19/27) had been bullied before they came to think about their gender identity.*"[12] They noted that "*adolescence is a period of identity formation* [identity formation, in general, not just with respect to gender]." But for most of the patients seeking "SRS", "*gender dysphoria presented in the context of wider identity confusion, severe psychopathology and considerable*

---

[10] Richard P. Fitzgibbons, Philip M. Sutton, and Dale O'Leary, "The Psychopathology of "Sex Reassignment" Surgery Assessing Its Medical, Psychological, and Ethical Appropriateness," *The National Catholic Bioethics Quarterly* (Spring 2009): 97-125.

[11] Richard P. Fitzgibbons, "Transsexual attractions and sexual reassignment surgery: Risks and potential risks," *The Linacre Quarterly* 82.4 (2015): 337–350.

[12] Riittakerttu Kaltiala-Heino, Maria Sumia, Marja Työläjärvi et al., "Two years of gender identity service for minors: overrepresentation of natal girls with severe problems in adolescent development," *Child and Adolescent Psychiatry and Mental Health* 9:9 (2015): 1-9, DOI 10.1186/s13034-015-0042-y.

challenges in the adolescent development." Therefore, in the presence of these difficulties, they do not advise that "SRS" be used as treatment.

Giovanardi et al. examined attachment patterns of 95 patients with "Gender Dysphoria" along with 123 control patients by examining their personal histories of childhood trauma. [13]Attachment patterns are formed from the way we relate emotionally to our primary caregivers as infants. They are characterized, for example, by the way a child behaves when threatened. These patterns have been described as secure, anxious, avoidant, and disorganized depending on how the child reacts with the caregiver in various situations. It is believed that poor quality attachments that develop in childhood can be *"a risk factor for psychopathology later in life."* [14]

They found that 69% of those with "Gender Dysphoria" had experienced three or more forms of childhood relational trauma including: rejection, neglect, physical abuse, psychological abuse, and /or separation by one or both parents. Only 10% had experienced no relational trauma. In contrast, 83% of the control group had experienced less than three forms of relational trauma.[15]

---

[13] Guido Giovanardi, Roberto Vitelli, Carola Maggiora Vergano, et al., "Attachment Patterns and Complex Trauma in a Sample of Adults Diagnosed with Gender Dysphoria." *Frontiers in Psychology* 9 (February 2018): 1-13, Article 60. DOI: 10.3389/fpsyg.2018.00060.

[14] Kasia Kozlowska, Catherine Chudleigh, Georgia McClure, et al., "Attachment Patterns in Children and Adolescents With Gender Dysphoria." *Frontiers in Psychology* 11 (January 2021): 1-21, Article 582688. DOI: 10.3389/fpsyg.2020.582688.

[15] Giovanardi et al., "Attachment Patterns and Complex Trauma," 1.

Lemma, while stating that she does not believe in "*a pre-deter-mined aim to therapy with transgendered individuals,*" does recognize that psychotherapy is a very important component of treating them.[16] Importantly, she notes that transgender may mean different things to different people.

Churcher Clarke and Spiliadis, present 12 cases of adolescents who met the criteria for "Gender Dysphoria" and were intent on medical intervention.[17] However, "[o]*ver the course of psychosocial assessment, they came to understand their distress and its alleviation (at that particular point in time) differently and eventually chose not take a medical (hormonal) pathway and/or identified their gender identity as broadly aligned with their biological sex.*" Of great importance is that many of the young people needed longer than the "*3-6 sessions*" of psychological assessment recommended in the "*current GIDS protocol*" at their London clinic.

While he does not believe "Gender Dysphoria" is a mental illness, Spiliadis does believe in a psychotherapeutic approach, and uses what he calls the "*Gender Exploratory Model*" to help his

---

[16] Alessandra Lemma, "Trans-itory identities: some psychoanalytic reflections on transgender identities." The International Journal of Psychoanalysis. 99.5 (2018): 1089–1106. https://doi.org/10.1080/00207578.2018.1489710.

[17] Anna Churcher Clarke and Anastassis Spiliadis, "'Taking the lid off the box': The value of extended clinical assessment for adolescents presenting with gender identity difficulties." Clinical Child Psychology and Psychiatry 24.2 (2019): 338– 352. DOI: 10.1177/1359104518825288.

patients.[18] In this model, he enters into a dialogue with the patient to explore the "*intersection of [their] gender identity with other markers of broader identity and psychosocial development.*" He presents one case of a young male seeking to transition who decided against doing so after therapy using the model.

Similarly, Kozlowska et al. investigated the attachment patterns of 57 children who presented to their gender service with "Gender Dysphoria." [19] In "structured attachment interviews," they gathered information about "*adverse childhood experiences (ACEs), mental health diagnoses, and global level of functioning.*" They compared results with those from age- and sex-matched children in a non-clinical group and another group with mixed psychiatric disorders. Children with "Gender Dysphoria" were "*mostly classified into the at-risk attachment strategies,*" and "*had a high rate of unresolved loss and trauma compared to children in the non-clinical group.*" These effects were statistically significant at the $p < 0.001$ level. Attachment patterns of children with "Gender Dysphoria" differed significantly from children in the non-clinical group, but not from the children with mixed psychiatric disorders. Nearly 90% of the children with "Gender Dysphoria" "*also suffered from one or more comorbid mental health disorders.*"

D'Angelo et al. note that "["Gender Dysphoria"] *can present as a transient symptom that resolves spontaneously or in the context of*

---

[18] Anastassis Spiliadis, "Towards a Gender Exploratory Model: slowing things down, opening things up and exploring identity development." *Metalogos Systemic Therapy Journal* 35 (July 2019).

[19] Kasia Kozlowska, et al., "Attachment Patterns in Children," 1.

developmentally informed psychotherapeutic treatment." [20] They also take issue with the moniker given to "*non-'affirmative' psychotherapy for GD as 'conversion'* [therapy]," noting that therapeutic interventions aim to help patients understand the reasons for their discomfort and explore their rationale for transitioning. They state that using a pejorative name for such psychotherapy "*will reduce access to treatment alternatives for patients seeking non-biomedical solutions to their distress.*"

In Part One, I noted that Fisher et al.[21] present a case study of a patient with "*gender identity variations coinciding solely with psychotic episodes during schizoaffective disorder, bipolar type.*" In other words, the 35-year-old male patient experienced "Gender Dysphoria" **only** when he was also experiencing "*psychotic breaks of schizoaffective disorder, bipolar type.*" The patient was treated with Risperidone (a commonly prescribed medicine for schizophrenia and bipolar disorder) and valproic acid (which is also used for bipolar disorder). In addition, he was treated with individual and group therapy. Within 8 days, the patient desisted from his "Gender Dysphoria" and was discharged to his home.

Sinai and Sim present another strong argument for '*psychodynamic psychotherapy*' to help address "Gender Dysphoria" and note

---

[20] Roberto D'Angelo, Ema Syrulnik, Sasha Ayad, et al., "One Size Does Not Fit All: In Support of Psychotherapy for Gender Dysphoria." *Archives of Sexual Behavior* 50 (2021): 7–16. https://doi.org/10.1007/s10508-020-01844-2.

[21] Kristy A. Fisher, Samantha Scemla, et al., "Gender Dysphoria Versus Acute Psychosis: Can One Properly Diagnose Gender Dysphoria Solely During Acute Psychosis?" *HCA Healthcare Journal of Medicine* 3.3 (2022): 167-173.

that it is <u>not</u> the same as conversion therapy.[22] *They note that "psy-chotherapy is a process of shared decision making in which the thera-pist ("perceiver") guides the patient in exploration of their material but does not input their own beliefs or ideas."* They note the near absence of psychotherapy for "Gender Dysphoria" in Canada and the rapidly growing number of detransitioners who desist from their "Gender Dysphoria." Many of these did not have psychotherapy in their jour-ney to transition which might have saved them significant suffering.

All of the above authors make it clear that the goal of psychother-apy is *"to help individuals gain a deeper understanding of their dis-comfort with themselves, the factors that have contributed to their dis-tress, and their motivations for seeking transition."*[23] Often, this is enough to resolve their dysphoria.

Therefore, the first line of treatment for any transgender individ-ual must be sincere, open-ended psychological counseling to rule out issues associated with past traumas or childhood issues. This will have a much greater chance of success if the dysphoric individual understands that they are suffering from a mental illness. With the gender-affirming model, the patient will believe they truly are trapped in the wrong body. One can only imagine that this would lead to more discomfort, and they will not believe that psychother-apy could have any benefit. However, if they understand that they have a mental disorder, then like those suffering from other illnesses, they will desire to be cured.

---

[22] Joanne Sinai and Peter Sim, "Psychodynamic psychotherapy for gen-der dysphoria is not conversion therapy," *Journal of the Canadian Academy of Child and Adolescent Psychiatry* 33:2 (July 2024): 145-153.

[23] D'Angelo et al., "One Size Does Not Fit All," 7.

Special Considerations for Children

Zucker[24] and Zucker and Spitzer[25] make note of several studies showing the majority of children with "Gender Dysphoria" become comfortable with their natal gender by the time they reach adolescence and young adulthood. Zucker observed that 88% of the children with "Gender Dysphoria" in his studies desisted, compared with 2.2% in a study done much earlier by Green. Nevertheless, a large majority of the children became comfortable with their natal gender. They hypothesize that "...*clinical evaluation and subsequent therapeutic intervention during childhood may alter the natural history of...*" "Gender Dysphoria."

Drescher[26] also pointed out that most cases of "Gender Dysphoria" in children resolve themselves before they become adults.

Kaltiala-Heino et al. state that the fact that most children, even with severe "Gender Dysphoria," don't persist into adolescence indicates "[medical] *interventions are therefore **not warranted** in prepubertal children* [my emphasis]."[27]

---

[24] Kenneth J. Zucker, "Gender Identity Disorder in Children and Adolescents," *Annual Review of Clinical Psychology* 1 (2005): 467–92, DOI: 10.1146/annurev.clinpsy.1.102803.144050.

[25] Kenneth J. Zucker and Robert L. Spitzer. "Was The Gender Identity Disorder Of Childhood Diagnosis Introduced Into DSM-III As A Backdoor Maneuver To Replace Homosexuality? A Historical Note." *Journal of Sex and Marital Therapy* 31 (2005): 31-42.

[26] Jack Drescher, "Queer Diagnoses: Parallels and Contrasts in the History of Homosexuality, Gender Variance, and the Diagnostic and Statistical Manual." *Archives of Sexual Behavior* 39.2 (2010): 427-60.

[27] Kaltiala-Heino, et al., "Two years of gender identity service," 1.

More recently, Singh et al. reported on 139 boys referred for "Gender Dysphoria" who were reassessed after an average of 13 years from their first clinic visit.[28] At follow-up, 88% of the boys had desisted and only 12% had persisted in their "Gender Dysphoria."

Similarly, Bachmann et al. studied German health insurance data of patients between 5 and 24 years old. Their results showed that after 5 years of follow-up, less than 50% of the patients persisted in their "Gender Dysphoria."[29] and persistence rates in various age groups were between 27% and 50%.

Even the National Health Service in the United Kingdom notes that "*in many cases gender variant behaviour* [sic] *or feelings disappear as children reach puberty.*"[30]

At least some "Gender Dysphoria" in children appears to have a psychological etiology according to Coates and Person, who claimed that gender identity disorder in some children was associated with "*a high incidence of separation anxiety*, and that these associations were revealed in psychotherapy."[31] They note that this anxiety is

---

[28] Devita Singh, Susan Bradley, and Kenneth Zucker, "A Follow-Up Study of Boys With Gender Identity Disorder" *Frontiers in Psychiatry* 12:632784 (2021): 1-18.

[29] Christian Bachmann, Yulia Golub, Jakob Holstiege, and Falk Hoffman, "Gender Identity Disorders Among Young People in Germany: Prevalence and Trends, 2013-2022. An Analysis of Nationwide Routine Insurance Data." *Dtsch Arztebl Int* 121 (2024): 370-1.

[30] National Health Service of the United Kingdom, "Gender Dysphoria – Treatment," https://www.nhs.uk/conditions/gender-dysphoria/treatment/.

[31] Susan Coates and Ethel Spector Person, "Extreme Boyhood Femininity: Isolated Behavior or Pervasive Disorder?" *Journal of the American Academy of Child Psychiatry* 24 (1985): 702–709.

often the result of *"actual separation trauma or a distant, disturbed mother-child interaction."*

A key takeaway from these studies is that "Gender Dysphoria" in most children desists by adolescence.[32] [33] [34] [35] [36] [37] [38] [39] This is a critical finding that significantly impacts any consideration of gender affirmation for children.

Special Considerations for Adolescents

"Gender Dysphoria" in adolescents may have a more complex etiology since it occurs in the context of a time of enormous changes in the lives of humans – adolescence. This is also a time of great pressure from one's peers which could play a large role in "Gender Dysphoria" at this stage of development as observed by Kaltiala-Heino et al.[40]

Korte et al. point to the *"multifactorial pathological process"* involved in development of "Gender Dysphoria."[41] At this critical time of development *"psychological factors exert their effects in concert*

---

[32] Fitzgibbons, et al., "The Psychopathology of "Sex Reassignment," 97.

[33] Fitzgibbons, "Transsexual attractions," 337.

[34] Kaltiala-Heino, et al., "Two years of gender identity service," 1.

[35] Paul W. Hruz, Lawrence S. Mayer, and Paul R. McHugh, "Growing Pains: Problems with Puberty Suppression in Treating Gender Dysphoria," *The New Atlantis*, 52 (Spring 2017): 3-36.

[36] Lemma, "Trans-itory identities," 1089.

[37] Churcher Clarke, et al., "'Taking the lid off the box'," 338.

[38] Spiliadis, "Towards a Gender Exploratory Model."

[39] D'Angelo et al., "One Size Does Not Fit All," 7.

[40] Kaltiala-Heino, et al., "Two years of gender identity service," 1.

[41] Korte, et al., "Gender Identity Disorders," 834.

with biological, familial, and sociocultural ones." They also observed that all of the patients reported on in their paper had *"psychopatho-logical abnormalities that, in many cases, led to the diagnosis of addi-tional psychiatric disorders. As a rule, there were also major psycho-pathological abnormalities in their parents."*

As a result, Korte et al. offer the opinion that, *"development in-hibiting... or body altering... <u>hormone therapy should not be initiated before the patient's psychosexual development is complete</u>, in view of the current lack of scientific data on these forms of treatment...* [my emphasis]."

Zucker believes that "Gender Dysphoria" also has a greater like-lihood of persistence in this age group.[42] He hypothesizes that *"An additional clue comes from consideration of the concepts of develop-mental malleability and plasticity. It is possible, for example, that gen-der identity shows relative malleability during childhood, with a grad-ual narrowing of plasticity as the gendered sense of self consolidates as one approaches adolescence."*

What is Treatment? - Brain plasticity, Puberty Blockers, and Cross-Sex Hormones

Much of the psychological literature points to the plasticity of the brain throughout life. This may account for adult onset of some cases of "Gender Dysphoria" and other mental illnesses. To some in the psychological community this suggests taking one of two pharma-cological approaches depending on the age of the patient. After all, pharmacological agents have been shown to help in many areas of

---

[42] Zucker, "Gender Identity Disorder in Children," 467.

mental illness, for example, clinical depression, bipolar disorder, and others.

Puberty Blockers

One approach is to provide puberty blockers to prevent young children from entering puberty so that they have "...*time to explore their gender identity, without the distress of the developing secondary sex characteristics.*"[43]

In 2022, the U.S. Food and Drug Administration issued a warning about the risk of "*pseudotumor cerebri (idiopathic intracranial hypertension)*" for patients receiving gonadotropin-releasing hormone (GnRH) agonists, i.e., puberty blockers.[44] There is a legitimate "on-label" use for puberty blockers in cases of precocious puberty. That is when a child begins puberty at unusually early age. In those cases, puberty blockers have established efficacy and safety assessed by the FDA.

However, using puberty blockers to delay puberty for "Gender Dysphoria" is an "off-label" use. As of September 2023, the FDA has not established efficacy or safety for this use. That fact led a group of concerned physicians and organizations to file "Citizen Petitions" to

---

[43] Paul W. Hruz, Lawrence S. Mayer, and Paul R. McHugh, "Growing Pains: Problems with Puberty Suppression in Treating Gender Dysphoria," *The New Atlantis*, 52 (Spring 2017): 3-36.

[44] American Academy of Pediatrics, "Risk of pseudotumor cerebri added to labeling for gonadotropin-releasing hormone agonists," AAP News, https://publications.aap.org/aapnews/news/20636/Risk-of-pseudo-tumor-cerebri-added-to-labeling-for?searchresult=1.

the FDA calling for urgent action to help define long-term risks and outcomes of their use. [45]

Even the National Health Service in the United Kingdom advises caution noting:

1) *"Puberty blockers (gonadotrophin-releasing hormone ana-logues) are not available to children and young people for gen-der incongruence or gender dysphoria because there is not enough evidence of safety and clinical effectiveness."*

2) *These hormones cause some irreversible changes such as... breast development... [and] breaking or deepening of the voice..."*

3) *Long-term cross sex hormone treatment may cause temporary or even permanent infertility.*

4) *There is some uncertainty about the risks of long-term cross-sex hormone treatment.* [46]

Relative to claims that puberty-blockers are reversible, Hruz et al. note the lack of *"... controlled clinical trials comparing the out-comes of puberty suppression to the outcomes of alternative therapeutic approaches."* They also report that *"there are reasons to suspect that*

---

[45] Jay T. Allen, Miriam Grossman, Patrick Hunter, et al., "Action Ur-gently Needed to Address Off-Label Use of Puberty Blockers in Children," https://downloads.regulations.gov/FDA-2023-P-3767-0001/attachment_1.pdf.

[46] National Health Service of the United Kingdom, "Gender Dysphoria – Treatment," online.

the treatments could have negative consequences for neurological development," citing a Scottish study. [47]

McPherson and Freedman reanalyzed data from an uncontrolled clinical study in the UK which involved 44 participants, aged 12 to 15 years old who were diagnosed with "Gender Dysphoria," and who were receiving Triptorelin, a gonadotropin releasing hormone (GnRH) agonist as a puberty blocker.[48] Because the original study had no controls, the authors assessed *"Reliable and Clinically Significant Change"* in the patients by comparing the CBCL and YSR at 12, 24, and 36 months follow up. The CBCL (Child Behavioral Checklist – Parent report) and YSR (Youth self-report) are established protocols for assessing general psychopathology in youth.[49] [50] [51] The authors found that the majority of the patients receiving puberty

---

[47] Hruz et al., "Growing Pains," 3.

[48] Susan McPherson and David E.P. Freedman, "Psychological outcomes of 12-15-year-olds with gender dysphoria receiving pubertal suppression in the UK: assessing reliable and clinically significant change," *Journal of Sex & Marital Therapy* 50.3 (2024): 315-325, DOI: 10.1080/0092623X.2023.2281986.

[49] Thomas M. Achenbach and Leslie A. Rescorla, "Empirically Based and DSM-Oriented Assessment of Preschoolers for Pharmacotherapy and Other Interventions," *Child & Adolescent Psychopharmacology News* 6.5 (September 2001): CAPN 1-7.

[50] Thomas M. Achenbach and Leslie A. Rescorla, "Practical Applications of the Achenbach System of Empirically Based Assessment (ASEBA) for Ages 1.5 to 90+ Years," *Australian Council for Educational Research* (July 20024) https://research.acer.edu.au/ research_conferenceITU_2004/2.

[51] Thomas M. Achenbach and Leslie A. Rescorla, "Child Behavior Checklist," in *Assessing Children's Well-Being – A Handbook of Measures,* eds. Sylvie Naar-King, Deborah A. Ellis, Maureen A. Frey (Mahwah, NJ: Lawrence Erlbaum Associates, Inc., 2004), 68-72.

blockers experienced "*no reliable change in distress across time points*." Perhaps more importantly, for internalizing and externalizing problems, "*between 15% and 29% deteriorate*." For total problems measured, they observed "*higher proportions deteriorating (20%-34%).*"

Given the above, Hruz et al. caution "[whether] *puberty suppression is safe and effective when used for gender dysphoria remains unclear and unsupported by rigorous scientific evidence*."[52]

Cross-Sex Hormones

A second approach, which is for adolescents and adults, is to provide cross-sex hormones to make the patient look like the gender they believe they are.

While Drescher[53] and others in the APA are concerned with the "*potential harm from GICE* [Gender Identity Conversion Efforts]," they do not seem to be at all concerned about injecting massive doses of steroids into patients, for long periods of time, in order to overcome their bodies' natural hormone levels. This seems to violate the physician's first principle to "Do No Harm." In fact, numerous studies have highlighted the risks of large doses of hormones. For example, Helzlsouer et al.[54] studied serum samples from over 20,000 women

---

[52] Hruz et al., "Growing Pains," 3.

[53] Drescher, "Queer Diagnoses," 427.

[54] Kathy J. Helzlsouer, Anthony J. Alberg, Gary B. Gordon, et al., "Serum Gonadotropins and Steroid Hormones and the Development of Ovarian Cancer," *Journal of the American Medical Association* 274.24 (1995): 1926-1930, DOI:10.1001/jama.1995.03530240036037.

in one Maryland County. *"The results suggest that women with ...high androgen levels have an increased risk of ovarian cancer."*

Similarly, Hage et al. reported on the occurrence of ovarian cancer in two female-to-male transsexuals.[55] They noted that *"Long-term exposure to increased levels of endogenous and exogenous androgens is hypothesized to constitute an additional risk factor in transsexuals as it has been associated with ovarian epithelial cancer."*

Mueller and Gooren found adenomas, breast cancer, and prostate cancer in male-to-female transsexuals receiving estrogen. They also observed breast carcinoma and several cases of ovarian cancer in female-to-male transsexuals receiving treatment with testosterone.[56] They noted that the probability of hormone-related tumors likely increases with the amount of time they are administered and age of the patients.

Other authors have also seen increased risk of cancers associated with prolonged hormone treatments. In a population-based, matched cohort study of transsexuals who underwent sex "reassignment" surgery, Dhejne et al.[57] reported *"cause-specific risk of death from neoplasms"* was increased by a factor of two (with *"borderline*

---

[55] J. J. Hage, J. J. M. L. Dekker, R. B. Karim, et al., "Ovarian Cancer in Female-to-Male Transsexuals: Report of Two Cases," *Gynecologic Oncology* 76 (2000): 413–415, DOI:10.1006/gyno.1999.5720.

[56] Andreas Mueller and Louis Gooren, "Hormone-related tumors in transsexuals receiving treatment with cross-sex hormones," *European Journal of Endocrinology* 159 (2008): 197–202, DOI: 10.1530/EJE-08-0289.

[57] Cecilia Dhejne, Paul Lichtenstein, Marcus Boman, et al., "Long-Term Follow-Up Of Transsexual Persons Undergoing Sex Reassignment Surgery: Cohort Study In Sweden." PLoS ONE 6.2 (February 2011): 1-8, E16885.

statistical significance" because of the small number of subjects). Cancers observed included lung, tongue, pharynx, pancreas and liver.

In a large study of nearly 5,000 transgender patients, Getahun et al. observed nearly 4-fold "*increases in VTE* [venous thromboembolism] *and ischemic stroke rates among transfeminine persons*" relative to their cisgender controls.[58]

Kaltiala and other researchers in Finland found that 90 percent of their patients were girls aged 15 to 17 years old, and that "*the vast majority presented with severe psychiatric conditions.*"[59] She notes that "*there is no mechanism by which high doses of hormones resolve [any] underlying mental health condition.*" In the end, Kaltiala and other physicians in different countries began to see that the patients they were treating with hormone therapy "*were not thriving. Instead, their lives were deteriorating.*"

An Aside Regarding Same-Sex Hormones

In one of the largest studies of its kind with almost 17,000 women subjects, Wassertheil-Smoller, et al. reported that the "*Women's Health Initiative (WHI) trial of estrogen plus progestin vs placebo was stopped early, after a mean 5.6 years of follow-up, because the overall*

---

[58] Darios Getahun, Rebecca Nash, W. Dana Flanders, et al., "Cross-sex Hormones and Acute Cardiovascular Events in Transgender Persons," *Annals of Internal Medicine* 169.4 (August 21, 2018): 205-213.

[59] Riittakerttu Kaltiala, "Gender-Affirming Care Is Dangerous. I Know Because I Helped Pioneer It," *The Free Press*, October 23, 2023, https://www.thefp.com/p/gender-affirming-care-dangerous-finland-doctor.

health risks of hormone therapy exceeded its benefits."[60] In fact, it was terminated 3 years before its planned completion date because *"its harmful effects outweighed its benefits."* Among the harmful effects was a *"...41% increase in locally adjudicated strokes over 5.2 years compared with women in the placebo group."* It should be noted that the hormones used in this study on women were **same-sex hormones**, not in the context of a "Gender Dysphoria" study.

Reporting on the same trial Heiss et al. observed that a *"greater risk of fatal and nonfatal malignancies occurred after the intervention and the global risk index was 12% higher in women randomly assigned to receive* [estrogen and progestin] *compared with placebo."*[61]

Therefore, it's clear that **even same-sex hormones can have negative effects** when used over long periods of time.

Some say that cross-sex hormone therapy is effective and that proves it is the treatment of choice. For example, apparently ignoring the health risks, Colizzi et al. [62] state that since hormone therapy induces changes in body features and shape, patients with "Gender Dysphoria" *"have been reported to experience a reduction in self-*

---

[60] Sylvia Wassertheil-Smoller, Susan Hendrix, Marian Limacher, et al., "Effect of Estrogen Plus Progestin on Stroke in Postmenopausal Women - The Women's Health Initiative: A Randomized Trial," *Journal of the American Medical Association* 289.20 (2003): 2673-2684, DOI:10.1001/jama. 289.20.2673.

[61] Gerardo Heiss, Robert Wallace, Garnet L. Anderson, et al., "Health Risks and Benefits 3 Years After Stopping Randomized Treatment With Estrogen and Progestin," *Journal of the American Medical Association* 299.9 (2008): 1036-1045, DOI:10.1001/jama.299.9.1036.

[62] Marco Colizzi, Rosalia Costa, Orlando Todarello, "Dissociative symptoms in individuals with gender dysphoria: Is the elevated prevalence real?" *Psychiatry Research* 226.1 (30 March 2015): 173-180.

reported distress." Similarly, Khorashad et al found that own-body perception changes favorably with cross-sex hormones.[63]

Nevertheless, just because a treatment reduced the psychological distress in a patient, doesn't mean that you have cured the illness because you don't know what really caused the disorder in the first place. One can only claim victory if one addresses the illness. For example, if I provide a massive dose of ibuprofen to a patient with chest pains, they may feel better, but they may still end up dying of a heart attack, because I have treated a symptom and not the disease.

In an overview of eating disorders, Murthy et al. noted that treatment of eating disorders does not just address the symptoms of the disorder, but must also address the *"…underlying psychological, interpersonal, and cultural forces that contributed to the eating disorder."*[64] Stapling the stomach of an anorexic to appease their desire to be slim, might seem to address the symptoms, but obviously is not a healthy approach.

In fact, Grant and Phillips showed that one treatment cannot be expected to fit all disorders.[65] In their study, Body Dysmorphic Disorder (BDD) and Anorexia Nervosa responded differently to treatment. A majority of patients with BDD improved with serotonin

---

[63] Behzad S. Khorashad1, Amirhossein Manzouri, Jamie D. Feusner, et al., "Cross-sex hormone treatment and own-body perception: behavioral and brain connectivity profiles," *Nature Scientific Reports* 11 (2021):2799.

[64] P N Murthy, P.P Dash, R Kumari, et al., "An Overview on Eating Disorders," Pharmacologyonline 3 (2009): 398-410.

[65] Jon E. Grant and Katharine A. Phillips, "Is Anorexia Nervosa a Subtype of Body Dysmorphic Disorder?

Probably Not, but Read On …," *Harvard Review of Psychiatry* 12.2 (2004): 123–126.

reuptake inhibitors; however, "...*BDD often responds well to cognitive-behavioral therapy, which has generally been less effective for anorexia.*"

What is Treatment? – Sex "Reassignment" Surgery

For some patients, hormone therapy is not enough. They want their bodies permanently altered to look like the opposite sex. "Gender Affirming Surgery," also known as Sex "Reassignment" Surgery ("SRS") surgery goes completely against nature by mutilating the body, removing healthy organs, and destroying the person's ability to continue the species by procreation. To add insult to injury, this "solution" requires never-ending, constant chemical bombardment with cross-sex hormones. As shown above, these chemicals are known to pose significant health risks, and are used just to retain an outward appearance that is biologically counterfeit.[66] [67] Nevertheless, even these extreme measures do not solve the problem.

For example, McHugh showed that there was no benefit to "SRS."[68] As former Psychiatrist-in-Chief at Johns Hopkins Medical Center, McHugh found these conclusions so compelling, that in 1979 all such surgeries at Johns Hopkins Medical Center were halted.

---

[66] Jack Drescher, "Controversies in Gender Diagnoses," *LGBT Health* 1.1 (2013): 1-5, DOI: 10.1089/lgbt.2013.1500.

[67] National Health Service of the United Kingdom, "Gender Dysphoria – Treatment," online.

[68] Paul R. McHugh, "Surgical Sex: Why We Stopped Doing Sex Change Operations." *First Things* 11 (2004): 34-38.

As discussed earlier, Reiner and Gearhart examined the limits of brain plasticity by studying 16 children who were born genetically male but had severe structural issues with the penis.[69] Fourteen of these children were assigned female at birth and had surgery to make their bodies resemble female anatomy. They were treated as girls thereafter by their parents. Nevertheless, Reiner and Gearhart found that 8 of the 14 declared themselves to be male later on in life. They noted that *"the sexual behavior and attitudes of all 16 subjects reflected male-type characteristics."*

Levine and Solomon reported that two of their 10 patients have had persistent, significant regrets about their transitions.[70] They further note that while *"...this rhetoric sounds remarkably certain about the long-term value of gender transition, hormones, and sex reassignment surgery in improving the lives of those with Gender Identity Disorder (GID), it is not."* They point out that careful studies with *"sophisticated follow-up... are lacking."*

Dhejne et al.[71] found that transexuals had three times the risk of psychiatric hospitalizations **after surgery** than control groups! They observed, *"substantially higher rates of overall mortality, death from cardiovascular disease and suicide, suicide attempts, and psychiatric*

---

[69] William G. Reiner and John P. Gearhart, "Discordant Sexual Identity in Some Genetic Males with Cloacal Exstrophy Assigned to Female Sex at Birth," *The New England Journal of Medicine* 350.4 (January 22, 2004): 333-341.

[70] Stephen B. Levine and Anna Solomon, "Meanings and Political Implications of "Psychopathology" in a Gender Identity Clinic: A Report of 10 Cases." *Journal of Sex and Marital Therapy* 35.1 (2008): 40-57.

[71] Cecilia Dhejne, "Long-Term Follow-Up," 1.

hospitalizations in sex-reassigned transsexual individuals compared to a healthy control population."

Mayer and McHugh after reviewing several studies on "SRS" outcomes conclude, "[the] *scientific evidence… suggests we take a skeptical view toward the claim that sex-reassignment procedures provide the hoped-for benefits or resolve the underlying issues that contribute to elevated mental health risks among the transgender population."* [72]

Fitzgibbons et al. and many other authors of the studies reviewed, acknowledge that no matter what is done, they haven't actually changed the person's sex. *"The publicly promoted goal of SRS is to transform a person of one sex into the other sex."* [73] Biologists will tell you that this is a physical impossibility because sex is determined by our genetic constitution which cannot be altered. *"Surgery can only create the appearance of the other sex."*

Therefore, by definition, the treatment has not addressed the illness. That is one of the points made by Cohen-Kettenis and Pfäfflin.[74] However, Cohen-Kettenis and Pfäfflin go on to state that the proper action is to change the DSM criteria, instead of admitting that the correct solution is not surgical but is psychiatric.

---

[72] Lawrence S. Mayer and Paul R. McHugh, "Sexuality and Gender: Findings from the Biological, Psychological, and Social Sciences." *The New Atlantis* 50 (Fall 2016): 10–143.

[73] Fitzgibbons, et al., "The Psychopathology of "Sex Reassignment" Surgery" 97.

[74] Peggy T. Cohen-Kettenis and Friedemann Pfäfflin, "The DSM Diagnostic Criteria for Gender Identity Disorder in Adolescents and Adults," *Archives of Sexual Behavior* 39.2 (2009): 499-513, DOI 10.1007/s10508-009-9562-y.

However, when adding the findings with respect to the un-changed psychological condition of patients after "SRS," it clearly argues against the use of "SRS" to "treat" "Gender Dysphoria."

Discussion

The recent HHS study summarized the dangers of a gender-affirming model for treatment of "Gender Dysphoria."[75] They noted, "[t]*hese interventions carry risk of significant harms including infertility/sterility, sexual dysfunction, impaired bone density accrual, adverse cognitive impacts, cardiovascular disease and metabolic disorders, psychiatric disorders, surgical complications, and regret. Meanwhile, systematic reviews of the evidence have revealed deep uncertainty about the purported benefits of these interventions.*"

For D'Angelo et al., "*...it is self-evident that the least-invasive treatment options should be pursued before progressing to more risky and irreversible interventions. To the extent that psychological treatments can help an individual obtain relief from GD without undergoing body-altering interventions, ensuring access to these interventions* [(psychotherapy)] *is not only* ethical *and* prudent *but also essential* [my emphases]."[76]

For many reasons, "gender-affirming treatment" must be considered unethical at best, criminal at worst.[77] Such treatment goes

---

[75] U.S. Department of Health and Human Services (hereafter, HHS), "Treatment for Pediatric Gender Dysphoria - Review of Evidence and Best Practices" (2025) https://opa.hhs.gov/gender-dysphoria-report.

[76] D'Angelo et al., "One Size Does Not Fit All," 12.

[77] Fitzgibbons, "Transsexual attractions," 337.

against what mainstream medicine would prescribe for any other condition. It mutilates or destroys otherwise healthy tissues. It does not do what it claims to do in that it does not change the sex of a patient to that of the opposite sex. It relegates the patient, among other harms, to a lifetime of cross-sex hormones whose toxicity has been demonstrated by many researchers.

For children, "gender-affirming treatment" addresses an issue from which the vast majority will desist. And it cannot be done with informed consent because children are not able to rationally understand the implications for their future lives.[78]

For adolescents with "Gender Dysphoria," the timing could not be worse. It is a period of immense physical, physiological, and psychological change even in individuals without "Gender Dysphoria." Given that the complex interrelationships of all these changes are not well understood, to meddle with one aspect is dangerous. The ethical approach must be to use therapy to understand the patient's development of their feelings and to help them understand where they came from. In many cases, it will be from adverse childhood experiences, poor attachments, or other psychological origins.

As I have shown, the literature is replete with cases of desistence from "Gender Dysphoria," often without intervention, but also after thoughtful psychoanalysis, and in at least one case pharmacological treatment aimed at the mind, not the body. Given the above examples, it is unconscionable that anyone, especially children, would be subjected to puberty suppression, cross-sex hormone therapy, and/or "SRS."

---

[78] Sinai and Sim, "Psychodynamic psychotherapy," 145.

Puberty suppression seems especially problematic. Many researchers, like Hruz at al. have noted "[puberty] *involves a myriad of complex, related, and overlapping physical processes, occurring at various points and lasting for various durations.*" [79] They go on to say, "*...whether blocking puberty is the best way to treat gender dysphoria in children remains far from settled and it should be considered not a prudent option with demonstrated effectiveness but a drastic and experimental measure.*" The fact that the use of puberty blockers to induce puberty suppression is considered off-label use means it has not been approved by the Food and Drug Administration. That also means that no one knows the effect of pausing/stopping the physical changes, meant to occur <u>during</u> puberty, on the other changes which nature has deemed <u>should occur simultaneously</u>. To say, as advocates do, that these changes are reversible, is at best wishful thinking and at worst a complete fabrication.

The authors of the recent HHS report note, "*the certainty of evidence is very low regarding the effect of PBs on GD..., improvement in mental health, and safety*"[80] and "*there is little data on what happens after treatment ends and the assumption that the effects of PBs are irreversible remains largely untested.*"[81]

Hruz et al. made an interesting observation relative to puberty suppression.[82] They note that "*...cross-gender identification apparently persists for virtually all who undergo puberty suppression* [which] *could indicate that these treatments increase the likelihood*

---

[79] Hruz et al., "Growing Pains," 4.

[80] HHS, "Treatment for Pediatric Gender Dysphoria," 87.

[81] Ibid., 88.

[82] Hruz et al., "Growing Pains," 10.

that the patients' cross-gender identification will persist." So, puberty suppression for "Gender Dysphoria" could be a self-fulfilling prophecy, ensuring that the child will persist in their dysphoric state.

There might be some rationale for using puberty blockers if they actually worked. However, as noted earlier, the McPherson and Freedman study showed little to no positive effect on participants stress and some deterioration in 15 to 34% of the subjects' mental health.[83] Similarly, the Cass Review, citing a University of York systematic review, noted there was *"no evidence that puberty blockers improve body image or dysphoria..."*[84]

The recent HHS report noted that since *"several studies have suggested continuation rates from PBs to CSH exceed 90%. The perception of PBs has shifted—from being seen as a reversible "pause button" to more like a "gas pedal" that accelerates medical transition."*[85] The authors also noted that the United Kingdom banned the use of puberty blockers except in clinical trials based on the Cass Review.[86]

Given the number of studies questioning the efficacy and safety of puberty blockers hormonal interventions in minors are now considered experimental or outright banned in Finland, Sweden, Denmark, Norway, Brazil, Chile, Alberta Canada, and Queensland Australia.[87]

---

[83] McPherson et al., "Psychological Outcomes," 319.

[84] Hilary Cass, "Independent review of gender identity services for children and young people: Final report." (2024) https://cass.independent-review.uk/home/publications/final-report/, 179.

[85] HHS, "Treatment for Pediatric Gender Dysphoria," 71.

[86] Ibid., 62.

[87] Ibid., 63.

With respect to cross-sex hormones, on the one hand, they can act on the body to make it seem to conform to how the patient feels. That does seem like a solution. On the other hand, if cross-sex hormones can be used to change the body, then why not use same-sex hormones to help make the patient's brain feel like the gender they were born? Given brain plasticity, there might be an effect on the brain that helps the patient feel more like their sex. Although this would have to be carefully tested, and even same-sex hormones can be dangerous as shown earlier, same-sex hormones should have far less deleterious effects on the patient population than cross-sex hormones. I don't know if this has been tried. While a mechanistic basis for benefit is not obvious,[88] it still seems an obvious approach to consider, and one which conforms to reality instead of affirming the pathology.

Perhaps more importantly, why would the psychiatric community not embrace psychological methods to bring mind and reality into sync? Some say there are no psychotherapies that work. If that's the case, researchers should try harder. Every problem has a solution if one is willing to work hard enough to find it.

In fact, as shown, there have been many reports in the literature of psychotherapeutic approaches that have been successful. Giovanardi et al.[89] and Kozlowska et al.[90] identified attachment patterns in children and adults that are highly correlated with "Gender

---

[88] Paul Hruz, Personal Communication, 2025.
[89] Giovanardi et al., "Attachment Patterns and Complex Trauma," 1.
[90] Kasia Kozlowska, et al., "Attachment Patterns in Children," 1.

Dysphoria." Di Ceglie[91] and Korte et al.[92] showed that in many cases gender issues due to early traumas or childhood difficulties, resolved with psychological counseling.

As discussed in the HHS Report, <u>there is clearly evidence showing benefits of psychotherapeutic approaches</u> in other mental health problems, including many of the co-morbidities associated with "Gender Dysphoria," and "*systematic reviews have found no evidence of adverse effects of psychotherapy in this context.*"[93]

This begs the question as to why hasn't the APA and mainstream psychology embraced these studies? One can only assume that political considerations have been interposed against the scientific realities and well-being of the patient population. The term "political" used here, is used in the sense of people with different agendas, not in the sense of political parties, per se. As I discussed in Part One, having served for over 30 years on many technical committees in the automotive industry, I am well aware of political influences on technical decisions. Political influences played a role in prolonging the development of a standard for the assessment of airbag noise for almost 25 years. I was the principal author and had to respond to many challenges brought by those who just didn't want another test to run. I saw similar challenges to crash test dummy development and acceptance. This politicization of psychology is an injustice to the patient population for whom the suffering is real and who deserve treatments in their best interest.

---

[91] Di Ceglie, "Gender Identity Disorder," 458.
[92] Korte, et al., "Gender Identity Disorders," 834.
[93] HHS, "Treatment for Pediatric Gender Dysphoria," 16 and 91.

Surgically removing organs of generation means that the patients will never be able to have their own children. Most of these surgeries contribute to life-long medical issues in those who receive them. As shown earlier Dhejne et al. (2011), found "...*substantially higher rates of overall mortality, death from cardiovascular disease and suicide, suicide attempts, and psychiatric hospitalizations in sex-reassigned transsexual individuals compared to a healthy control population.*" [94]

As D'Angelo noted, "*ensuring access to these* [therapeutic] *interventions is not only ethical and prudent but also essential.*"[95]

There are two ways one can view "Gender Dysphoria." In the first way, one could say that "the patient's body doesn't match their feelings." In the second way, one could say that "the patient's feelings don't match their body." In the first case, one would try to change the body to effect a cure. In the second case, one would try to change the feelings to effect a cure. Simple inspection tells us which of the two statements is objectively true. The other is totally subjective and, therefore, seems to be the better candidate for remediation. Just because hormone therapy makes some "Gender Dysphoria" patients feel better, doesn't mean that the correct psychological treatment wouldn't also make them feel better and at the same time spare their body the potentially damaging effects of hormones.

This lack of true leadership by the APA and others has worked its way into enacted legislation. Advocacy groups have spoken louder than clinicians and scientists forcing governments to cooperate with their ill-informed desires, at best, or their malicious intent, at worst. For example, Zucker was psychologist-in-chief at Toronto's Centre

---

[94] Cecilia Dhejne, "Long-Term Follow-Up," 1.
[95] D'Angelo et al., "One Size Does Not Fit All," 7.

for Addiction and Mental Health (CAMH) and head of its Gender Identity Service until an advocacy organization claimed his methods were out of step with those espoused by WPATH (World Professional Association for Transgender Health).[96] Zucker, a world expert in child psychology and "Gender Dysphoria," was then fired and his clinic closed.[97] And now, "[in] *Canada, psychological assessment prior to hormonal therapy is typically minimal*" because "[psychotherapy] *plays little or no role in the gender affirming model.*"[98]

Similarly, Minnesota has a law that allows minors from other states to travel there for "gender-affirming" procedures irrespective of their parents' wishes.[99] It is well accepted that children and adolescents are not mature enough to make important life-changing decisions. This is why there are laws establishing minimum ages for driving, voting, drinking, etc. It is unethical at best, criminal at worst, to allow children and adolescents to give "informed consent," especially when they are suffering from a mental disorder.

Unfortunately, the organization claiming to set the standards of care for people with "Gender Dysphoria" is little more than an

---

[96] Wikipedia, "Kenneth Zucker," https://en.wikipedia.org/wiki/Kenneth_Zucker#:~:text=Citing%20a%20review%20by%20two,was%20found%20to%20be%20false.

[97] Mayer and McHugh, "Sexuality and Gender," 10.

[98] Sinai and Sim, "Psychodynamic psychotherapy," 145-153.

[99] Caroline Downey, "Tim Walz Signed Bill Making Minnesota a Sanctuary State for Child Sex-Changes," National Review, August 6, 2024, https://www.nationalreview.com/news/tim-walz-signed-bill-making-minnesota-a-sanctuary-state-for-child-sex-changes/#:~:text=Dubbed%20the%20Trans%20Refuge%20Bill,medical%20practitioners%20who%20provide%20it.

advocacy group. [100] "*WPATH is neither solely a professional body...
nor does it represent the 'world' view... [as] there is no global agreement on best practice* [for treating "Gender Dysphoria"]." Files leaked
from the organization show acknowledgement by high level members of the organization of permanent sexual disfunction from puberty blockers and possible liver cancers from hormone treatments.
This is addressed at length in the HHS Report.[101] Of great concern is
that the American Academy of Pediatrics, an organization one would
expect to advocate for the health and safety of children, actually
threatened to oppose WPATH's Standards of Care version 8 unless
lower age limits were removed! [102]

To make matters worse, the HHS report shows "*the best available
evidence indicates that PBs, CSH, and surgery have not been shown to
improve mental health outcomes.*"[103] Similarly, the "*best available evidence, along with a risk/benefit analysis and precautionary approach
ethically appropriate to pediatrics*" shows that pediatric medical transitions "*do not provide benefits proportionate to its harms.*"[104]

Finally with respect to children the HHS Report states, "*It is not
ethical to subject adolescents to hormonal and surgical interventions
used in [Pediatric Medical Transitions], even in a research trial, until*

---

[100] Hannah Barnes, "Why disturbing leaks from US gender group
WPATH ring alarm bells in the NHS," *The Guardian* March 9, 2024,
https://www.theguardian.com/commentisfree/2024/mar/09/disturbing-
leaks-from-us-gender-group-wpath-ring-alarm-bells-in-nhs?CMP=
share_btn_url.

[101] HHS, "Treatment for Pediatric Gender Dysphoria," Chapter 10.

[102] Ibid., 179.

[103] HHS, "Treatment for Pediatric Gender Dysphoria," 221.

[104] Ibid., 236.

and unless the state of the evidence suggests a favorable risk/benefit profile for the studied intervention, and the researchers have well-grounded confidence that the foreseeable 'risks and burdens have been adequately assessed and can be satisfactorily managed.'"[105] I would argue that the same applies to adult patients.

Psychological Counseling or "Reparative Therapy"?

D'Angelo et al. show how advocacy groups have used flawed studies, promoted in media campaigns, to influence government decision makers who are not specialists and therefore cannot easily make informed decisions.[106] The authors noted that there was no scientific debate about one flawed study, in particular, and that *"all of the letters written to the Editor of JAMA Psychiatry, many by respected academics and clinicians who outlined the serious problems in the study, have been rejected."* The flawed study demonized psychotherapy for "Gender Dysphoria" as "conversion therapy," which is used as a pejorative term by transgender activists. The advocates will not allow any attempt to actually help those with "Gender Dysphoria" – affirmation is their god.

In contrast to his discourse about labeling and stigmatizing those with "Gender Dysphoria," that is exactly what Drescher (2010) does to the researchers who do not agree with his beliefs. He puts all attempts to use psychological counseling to help those with "Gender Dysphoria" into the heading of "Reparative Therapy," which has also come to be a pejorative term for Gender Identity Conversion Efforts

---

[105] Ibid., 239.

[106] Roberto D'Angelo, et al., "One Size Does Not Fit All," 7.

(GICE). His bias is clear in the later statement *"This author believes a more detailed and scholarly study of* **potential harm** *from GICE and how that may compare with SOCE seems worthwhile* [my emphasis]." Note the lack of balance in this statement, in contrast to a statement such as, "This author believes a more detailed and scholarly study of **the efficacy of** GICE and how that may compare with SOCE seems worthwhile." Here the word efficacy does not imply a foregone conclusion but is open to scientific facts. It is clear that Drescher does not believe "Gender Dysphoria" is a psychological disorder, and he takes the unprecedented approach in his paper of calling into question the integrity of the researchers who publish views contrary to what he believes (pg. 451). This is an *ad hominem* attack instead of a discussion of facts and has no place in scientific discourse.

As noted earlier in this work, and also in the HHS Report, the fact that psychotherapeutic approaches are effective for a wide range of mental disorders, including many of the co-morbidities of "Gender Dysphoria," is strongly suggestive of anticipated benefit for patients with "Gender Dysphoria."[107]

Conclusions to Part Two

Clearly, for any psychotherapy to work, the patient must want to be cured. In an environment where the professionals needed to treat the patients are engaged in public debate about whether the patients are really ill, one cannot expect that the patients will embrace treatment.

---

[107] HHS, HHS, "Treatment for Pediatric Gender Dysphoria," 257.

Allowing mental disorder of a small percentage of the population to cause the majority to change their way of life is immoral at best, lunacy at worst. Allowing people of the opposite sex to share bathrooms, changing rooms, and dormitories, has already led to multiple cases of sexual assault. Allowing transsexual women to compete in women's sports when clear biological differences are present that allow their natal male bodies to dominate is an injustice to women in sports everywhere.

Proposed Actions from Part Two:

- Given the evidence that does exist for successful psychotherapy, all efforts should be directed to helping the mind explore the reasons for their feelings and ultimately to accept the reality of the body.

  o If there is no agreement on which therapies, if any, are effective, then large scale clinical research should be undertaken to find some that are. By continuing to consider cross-sex hormone treatments and sex "reassignment" surgeries to be therapies, the psychiatric, psychological, and medical professions have abandoned Hippocrates mandate to "do no harm."[108]

---

[108] Hippocrates, "Of the Epidemics", Section II, Second Constitution, Number 5, from https://classics.mit.edu/Hippocrates/epidemics.1.i.html.

- In the meantime, other methods (pharmaceutical and psychological) should be used to reduce the patient's discomfort and distress (e.g., anti-anxiety meds, anti-depressants, etc.)
- Research into pharmacological methods to bring the mind into order again should be investigated.
- This author does not have historical information as to why cross-sex hormone treatments were considered appropriate. However, there is evidence that cross-sex hormones reinforce the dysphoria. Therefore, the question of whether any research has been done into using same-sex hormones to work in synergy with brain plasticity and to help change the mind into realizing its physical reality. This hypothesis would be especially strong if data shows that children who desist do so around the time of puberty which would be a time of surging endogenous hormones.

"Gender Dysphoria" is clearly real to the patients who experience it. Otherwise, who would be willing to risk losing loved ones by transitioning, or who would undergo painful life-altering surgeries? Patients are suffering. The key question is what should be done to help them? The leaders of the psychiatric community, at the prompting of perhaps well-meaning advocacy groups, most of whom are not medical or psychiatric professionals, and with the consent of governments interested more in political correctness than their citizens, have engaged in the largest-scale scientific experiment on human subjects in history. And they have done this without informed consent. In fact, the patients being studied have not been told the true risks and the true nature of their "treatment", viz, that it is entirely experimental and, in many cases, irreversible. It's impossible to give informed consent without that information. This is simply unethical behavior.

PART THREE

A CATHOLIC PERSPECTIVE
ON "GENDER DYSPHORIA"

Abstract

In this third part," I have sought to develop a Catholic perspective using the Sacred Scriptures, the Catechism of the Catholic Church, and Magisterial documents. I also address the attempt by human beings to reject what God has made and to refashion themselves in their own image, the inappropriateness of taking steps to transition children, and the negative effects of transitioning on the individual and their families. I discuss spiritual warfare, the importance of compassion for those afflicted by this disorder, and a call for action by the Catholic Church and community.

Introduction

As Saint Pope Paul VI stated in his much-discussed Encyclical Letter, Humanae Vitae, "...*man has made stupendous progress in the domination and rational organization of the forces of nature, such that he tends to extend this domination to his own total being: to the body, to psychical life, to social life...*"[1] This prophetic statement is especially true today as humans seek to change their God-given bodies into those of the opposite sex. He went on to say, "*Such questions*

---

[1] Paul VI, *Humanae Vitae* (July 25, 1968), n.2.

[require] *from the teaching authority of the Church a new and deeper reflection upon the principles of moral teaching... a teaching founded on the natural law, illuminated and enriched by divine revelation."* While originally stated in the context of marriage, this is no less true for the issue of "Gender Dysphoria."[2] The Pope noted that Jesus gave to St. Peter and the Apostles authority, guardianship, and the job of authentic interpretation of moral law and natural law which is "*an expression of the will of God.*"

In his encyclical Caritas in Veritate, Pope Bendict XVI said, "*To defend the truth, to articulate it with humility and conviction, and to bear witness to it in life are... exacting and indispensable forms of charity. Charity, in fact, 'rejoices in the truth' (1 Cor 13:6)"*[3] After noting that the Church's social doctrine is based on charity, he went on to say, "*Only in truth does charity shine forth, only in truth can charity be authentically lived. Truth is the light that gives meaning and value to charity... Without truth, charity degenerates into sentimentality. Love becomes an empty shell, to be filled in an arbitrary way. In a culture without truth... [it] falls prey to contingent subjective emotions and opinions, the word "love" is abused and distorted, to the point where it comes to mean the opposite.*"[4]

There are those in society who claim the only way to love a person suffering from "Gender Dysphoria" is to affirm their desire to change their body into that of the opposite sex. In Part One, I

---

[2] I will continue to capitalize the term "Gender Dysphoria" and put it in quotation marks in this paper unless it is used in a direct quote. In that case, I will follow the style of the paper being cited.

[3] Benedict XVI, *Caritas in Veritate*, (June 29, 2009), n. 1.

[4] Benedict XVI, *Caritas in Veritate*, n. 3.

summarized the evidence leading to the unavoidable conclusion that the gender variance associated with "Gender Dysphoria," and therefore, the whole of "Gender Dysphoria" is a mental disorder. In Part Two, I examined the fraud of gender-affirming treatments and the availability of more rational alternatives. As will be discussed, "…*it is never compassionate to approve of efforts to identify as other than one's biological sex.*"[5] Not telling the truth to those who are clearly and really suffering with "Gender Dysphoria," is not charity, it is false compassion and contrary to all Catholic teaching.

In this part, I will seek to answer the question "How should I as a Catholic Christian view the issue of "Gender Dysphoria?" I will present an analysis of Church teaching and a summary of the published faith-based literature related to this topic.

Right at the start I will note that the faithful Catholic is obligated to use their properly formed conscience in matters of moral questions. When properly formed, our conscience can take into account the natural laws inscribed on our hearts by our loving God. These are knowable by right reason. For example, all societies acknowledge that murder is wrong. The 10 commandments are simply a record on stone of what God has already written in our hearts.

However, many people do not have properly formed consciences for a variety of reasons. Then, as a first step, they should seek counsel from their parish priest in areas of moral question. Yet, in some cases the priest may not be well-versed on a new or highly technical issue. In such cases, one of the positive aspects of the

---

[5] The Most Rev. Allen H. Vigneron, "*The Good News About God's Plan: A Pastoral Letter on the Challenges of Gender Identity*," (February26, 2024), 7.

internet in our modern society is that it has connected people with a plethora of resources for investigating Catholic teaching on many issues. Still some issues may be lacking in resources, and many websites have an inherent bias based on the website owner's agenda. There are, however, resources available within the Catholic sphere that are reliable. The faithful must use the knowledge and moral guidance that are present in, the Sacred Scriptures, the Catechism of the Catholic Church, the Magisterium of the Church (Papal documents and pastoral letters from the Pope and other Bishops), and other reputable resources to form their conscience to the best of their abilities.

Using this model, we can construct a reasonable view of "Gender Dysphoria" in light of Natural Law and Catholic teaching.

What Does Scripture Say About "Gender Dysphoria?"

The place to start with any moral dilemma for a Christian is Sacred Scripture. As one would imagine, the terms "Gender Dysphoria" and "Transsexual" do not appear in the Sacred Scriptures. There are, however, a number of statements that apply to the discussion. The most obvious statements addressing "Gender Dysphoria" come from Genesis:

- *"So, God created man in his own image, in the image of God he created him; male and female he created them."* [6]

---

[6] Catholic Biblical Association, (Great Britain) *The Holy Bible: Revised Standard Version, Catholic edition* (New York: National Council of Churches of Christ in the USA, 1994), Gen. 1:27.

- *"When God created man, he made him in the likeness of God. Male and female he created them..."*[7]

There is no uncertainty in these statements. They stand on their own merits without need of explanation. Jesus Himself, reinforced this teaching in the Gospels of Mark and Matthew when he said:

- *"But from the beginning of creation, 'God made them male and female.'"*[8]
- *"He answered, "Have you not read that he who made them from the beginning made them male and female..."*[9]

In a Pastoral Letter to his flock in the Archdiocese of Detroit, Archbishop Allen Vigneron explained the ramifications of these scripture passages. He noted, *"This creation account from the Book of Genesis is the "beginning" to which Jesus calls us to return, revealing the beautiful and foundational truths about the human person. First among these truths is that we are not byproducts or accidents; we are created. To be created is to be chosen, willed, and intended* [emphasis added]." Since we are willed by God into existence, He must have willed that we be male or female. Archbishop Vigneron continues, *"Sex is assigned, not by a doctor or the individual, but genetically and biologically by God in the act of creation."*[10]

---

[7] Ibid (Genesis 5:1–2).

[8] Ibid. (Mark 10:6).

[9] Ibid. (Matthew 19:4).

[10] The Most Rev. Allen H. Vigneron, *"The Good News About God's Plan,"* pgs. 2-3.

A statement of God's intentions in the establishment of the complementary nature of man and woman can also be found in Genesis. *"28And God blessed them, and God said to them, "Be fruitful and multiply..."*[11] Thus, it was God's intent for male and female to be co-creators with him of the human race, something only possible if they have complementary sexual organs and both are sexually fertile and capable of "being fruitful and multiplying." This manner of creation is also the first Revelation of God's plan for the human family.

The next selection from Sacred Scripture that bears on the issue of "Gender Dysphoria" is again taken from the Old Testament. It comes from Deuteronomy 22:5 which states *"A woman shall not wear anything that pertains to a man, nor shall a man put on a woman's garment; for whoever does these things is an abomination to the LORD your God."* [12] This statement makes it pretty clear that God does not intend for there to be any confusion as to who is a man and who is a woman. Again, He does not leave any room for misinterpretation.

The New Testament is less direct about references that would address "Gender Dysphoria." In particular, the writings of St. Paul refer to two types of men, malakoi (μαλακοὶ) and arsenenokoitais (ἀρσενοκοίτης) which the RSV Translation calls "sexual perverts" and the NASB calls "effeminate men" and "male homosexuals," respectively. Both terms denote homosexuals, one in a male role and the other in a female role. In the King James Version of the Bible, the translation reads *"Know ye not that the unrighteous shall not*

---

[11] Ibid. (Genesis 1:28).

[12] Ibid. (Deuteronomy 22:5).

inherit the kingdom of God? Be not deceived: neither fornicators, nor idolaters, nor adulterers, nor effeminate (μαλακοὶ), *nor abusers of themselves with mankind* (ἀρσενοκοίτης) ..." Men for whom "Gender Dysphoria" is a subconscious coping mechanism for same-sex attraction would likely fall under this category.[13] [14]

Another critical piece of information to be gleaned from Sacred Scripture is that God willed there to be an order to the universe in His Creation, and this order extends to human nature.[15] As stated by the Committee on Doctrine of the United States Conference of Catholic Bishops, "*A crucial aspect of the order of nature created by God is the body-soul unity of each human person.*" We are called to respect this order created and willed by God. We'll come back to this point.

Does Anything in the Catechism Expressly Address "Gender Dysphoria?"

As in the case of Sacred Scripture, the terms "Gender Dysphoria" and "Transsexual" do not appear anywhere in the Catechism of the

---

[13] Kenneth J. Zucker, and Robert L. Spitzer. "Was The Gender Identity Disorder Of Childhood Diagnosis Introduced Into DSM-III As A Backdoor Maneuver To Replace Homosexuality? A Historical Note." *Journal of Sex & Marital Therapy* 31 (2005): 31-42.

[14] Kenneth J. Zucker, "Gender Identity Disorder in Children and Adolescents," *Annual Review of Clinical Psychology* 1 (2005): 467–92, DOI: 10.1146/annurev.clinpsy.1.102803.144050.

[15] United States Conference of Catholic Bishops Committee on Doctrine, "*Doctrinal Note on the Moral Limits to Technological Manipulation of the Human Body,*" (March 20, 2023), n.2, 3, 4.

Catholic Church.[16] The Catechism cannot and does not contain information on every possible moral conflict and cannot predict what new moral conflicts will arise in the future. Then, how is a faithful and responsible Catholic to know what authentic Church teaching is relative to this subject? As it turns out, there is still information to be found in the Catechism that is pertinent to the subject even though those terms don't appear. According to the Catechism of the Catholic Church:

- **CCC 364** - *"man … is obliged to regard his body as good and to hold it in honor since God has created it."* [17]
- **CCC 355** - *"God created man in his own image… male and female he created them."*[18]
- **CCC 362 and 364** - "[The human person is] *at once corporeal and spiritual,"*[19] [and] *"animated by a spiritual soul."*[20]
- **CCC 365** - *"…spirit and matter, in man, are not two natures united, but rather their union forms a single nature."*[21]
- **CCC 366** - "[The] *Church teaches that every spiritual soul is created immediately by God—it is not 'produced' by the parents."*[22]

---

[16] Catholic Church, *Catechism of the Catholic Church*, 2nd Ed. (Washington, DC: United States Catholic Conference, 2000). Hereafter, CCC.

[17] CCC 364.

[18] Catholic Biblical Association, The Holy Bible, Gen. 1:27, and CCC 355.

[19] CCC 362.

[20] CCC 364.

[21] CCC 365.

[22] CCC 366.

- **CCC 369** - *"Man and woman have been created, which is to say, willed by God… in their respective beings as man and woman. 'Being man' or 'being woman' is a reality which is good and willed by God…. In their 'being-man' and 'being-woman,' they reflect the Creator's wisdom and goodness."*[23]
- **CCC 2333** - *"Everyone, man and woman, should acknowledge and accept his sexual identity."*[24]
- **CCC 2297** - *"Except when performed for strictly therapeutic medical reasons, directly intended amputations, mutilations, and sterilizations performed on innocent persons are against the moral law."*[25]

In the citations above, it is clear that there is no other option besides male or female in God's creation, and each human is to regard his/her body as good.

Papal Statements that are Relevant to Gender Dysphoria

As head of the Church and leader of the Magisterium, the Pope's opinion of moral issues is of the utmost importance.

Pope Pius XII's address, mentioned earlier, was to the "First International Congress of Histopathology of the Nervous System."[26] The meeting was one of medical professionals reviewing new findings allowed by modern technologies and methods. The Pope noted

---

[23] CCC 369.

[24] CCC 2333.

[25] CCC 2297.

[26] Pius XII, *Speech from Pope Pius XII*, Introduction, Para 2.

that he was not there to address the limits of the medical field, but rather, the *"limits of moral rights and duties."*

In his speech, Pope Pius XII noted that the *"'interest of the patient' provides in many cases the moral justification for the doctor's conduct."* However, *"the patient... is not the absolute master of himself, of his body, of his mind. He cannot therefore freely dispose of himself as he pleases."* The patient is the user, not the owner of his/her body and *"does not have unlimited power to perform acts of destruction or mutilation of an anatomical or functional nature."*[27] There are moral limits to the patients actions which include that the patient can only dispose of individual body parts, or mutilate them if doing so will repair serious damage, and/or ensure the existence of the individual (i.e., keep them from dying).

Gaudium et Spes (1965), a document of the Second Vatican Council promulgated by St. Pope Paul VI, states *"Though made of body and soul, man is one... For this reason man is not allowed to despise his bodily life, rather he is obliged to regard his body as good and honorable since God has created it and will raise it up on the last day."*[28]

In Humanae Vitae, St. Pope Paul VI went further. *"In relation to the tendencies of instinct and passion... [there is a] necessary dominion which reason and will must exercise over them."*[29] Although originally stated regarding marital intimate relations, this statement bears equally well with respect to feelings of any kind, such as

---

[27] Ibid. Section II, Para. 2 and 4.

[28] Paul VI, *Gaudium et Spes* (December 7, 1965), no.14.

[29] Paul VI, *Humanae Vitae*, n.10.

"Gender Dysphoria." Feelings must be subordinate to reason and morality.

After St. Paul's letter to the Romans (3:8), Paul VI says, "*In truth… it is not licit, even for the gravest reasons, to do evil so that good may follow therefrom.*"[30] Taken together with CCC 2297 above, this directly applies to sex "reassignment" surgery. CCC 2297 states that "*mutilations… on innocent persons are against the moral law.*" Paul VI gives insight as to why this prohibition exists a little further on in the document. He notes, "*…the Church is the first to praise and recommend the intervention of intelligence in a* [bodily] *function… but she affirms that this must be done with respect for the order established by God.*"[31] While originally written with respect to developing methods of preventing pregnancy, one can clearly apply this to "Gender Dysphoria" too. In other words, we do not have absolute dominion over our bodies, and to act as if we do, is an offense against God's sovereignty.[32] Therefore, although a person with "Gender Dysphoria" might consider it to be therapy, from guidance given by the Church, "SRS" would not be morally acceptable.[33]

In his theology of the body, Pope John Paul II explains how sex is not just an attribute of a human person but has a much deeper

---

[30] Paul VI, *Humanae Vitae*, n.14.

[31] Paul VI, *Humanae Vitae*, n.16.

[32] Fr. John Hardon, "Modern Catholic Dictionary," as cited by Catholic Culture website, https://www.catholicculture.org/culture/library/dictionary/index.cfm?id=35019.

[33] In this part, I will continue to use the term 'sex "reassignment" surgery' with "reassignment" in quotes, or "SRS" also in quotes, unless it is used in a direct quote. In that case, I will follow the style of the paper being cited.

meaning. "*Precisely the function of sex [that is, being male or female], which in some way is "constitutive for the person" (not only 'an attribute of the person'), shows how deeply man, with all his spiritual solitude, with the uniqueness and unrepeatability proper to the person, is constituted by the body as 'he' or 'she'.*"[34] By "constitutive to the person' the Holy Father means that sex is something without which a person would no longer be a person.

Of significance in the argument from philosophy, later in this document, is another teaching by Pope John Paul II. In Veritatis Splendor, he states, "*...the Church's teachings on the unity of the human person, whose rational soul is <u>per se et essentialiter</u> the form of his body. The spiritual and immortal soul is the principle of unity of the human being, whereby it exists as a whole - <u>corpore et anima unus</u> - as a person.*"[35]

Pope Benedict XVI made several statements as reported in the press, regarding "gender theory". In an address to the Roman Curia in December of 2012,[36] Pope (then Emeritus) Benedict stated "*People dispute the idea that they have a nature, given by their bodily identity, which serves as a defining element of the human being. They deny their nature and decide that it is not something previously given to them, but that they make it for themselves. According to the biblical creation account, being created by God as male and female pertains*

---

[34] John Paul II, (M. Waldstein, Trans.) *Man and woman He created them: A theology of the body* (Boston: Pauline Books & Media, 2006), 166.

[35] John Paul II, *Veritatis Splendor* (August 6, 1993), n. 48.

[36] Cited in Catholic Online article by Deacon Keith Fournier, "Is Transgenderism a Mental Disorder of a Right?" http://www.catholic.org/news/national/story.php?id=56646.

to the essence of the human creature. This duality is an essential as-pect of what being human is all about, as ordained by God."

In that same address, he added "*When the freedom to be creative becomes the freedom to create oneself, then necessarily the Maker himself is denied and ultimately man too is stripped of his dignity as a creature of God...*"

Similarly, Pope Francis stated ""*God has placed man and woman [at] the summit of creation and has entrusted them with the earth... The design of the Creator is written in nature.*" The Pope also com-pared gender theory to nuclear arms which can destroy an extraor-dinary number of human lives in an instant and so '...*does not rec-ognize the order of creation.*'"[37]

In his encyclical, *Laudato Si*, Pope Francis is even more direct.[38] "*The acceptance of our bodies as God's gift is vital... whereas thinking that we enjoy absolute power over our own bodies turns, often subtly, into thinking that we enjoy absolute power over creation. Learning to accept our body, to care for it and to respect its fullest meaning, is an essential element of any genuine human ecology. Also, valuing one's own body in its femininity or masculinity is necessary... In this way we can joyfully accept the specific gifts of another man or woman, the work of God the Creator, and find mutual enrichment.*"

Finally, in *Amoris Laetitia*, Pope Francis states that there is a no-tion that is rampant in today's society in which people "*confuse*

---

[37] Joshua J. McElwee, "Francis Strongly Criticizes Gender Theory, Comparing it to Nuclear Arms." *National Catholic Reporter*, February 13, 2015, http://ncronline.org/news/vatican/francis-strongly-criticizesgender-theory-comparing-nuclear-arms.

[38] Francis, *Laudatio Si* (May 24, 2015), n. 155.

genuine freedom with the idea that each individual can act arbitrarily as if there were no truths, values and principles to provide guidance, and everything were possible and permissible."[39]

Thus, the simple truth from Church teaching that God created us male and female remains a basic fact. Added to this is the fact that we are not free to do whatever we will with our bodies if it goes against the order of Creation given by God.

So, What Should the Church Teach about "Gender Dysphoria"

Argument from Philosophy

Some in the transgender world claim that they are female souls in male bodies or vice versa. This claim hearkens back to the heresy of Gnosticism which appeared around the end of the second century.[40] Gnostics considered human beings to be entrapped souls, not a union of spirit and matter. But that is fundamentally at odds with the basic tenets of Catholicism. As stated earlier, the Church teaches in the Catechism that, "…*spirit and matter, in man, are not two natures united, but rather their union forms a single nature.*"[41] The soul is the "*spiritual principle*" in man and without it, one would not be human. "*The body and soul come into existence together, in an individual human being at the time of conception. From the beginning of*

---

[39] Francis, *Amoris Lætitia* (March 19, 2016), n. 34.

[40] Fr. Robert Barron, "Bruce Jenner, The 'Shadow Council,' and St. Irenaeus" www.wordonfire.org 6/9/15.

[41] CCC 365.

his or her existence, the human person has a body that is sexually differentiated as male or female."[42]

Philosophically, there are two ways to look at this, a Thomistic view, and another view proposed by John D. Finley.[43]

According to the view of St. Thomas Aquinas, the human soul is spirit and not matter,[44] and sexual differentiation is intrinsic to matter and not to spirit. Therefore, in this view the claim that there is a male or female soul at all is *prima facie* false.

However, within St. Thomas' view, if one was to accept that souls are sexually differentiated, the idea that God would put a female soul into a male body would lead to one of several conclusions. First, that God made a mistake. However, by definition, God cannot and does not make mistakes. Another possible conclusion would be that God intentionally put a female soul into a male body. However, because He is the only Creator of souls, given the pain and confusion that we see in those who experience "Gender Dysphoria," this would be the same as saying, God intentionally caused pain and suffering. We can say this because if God intentionally put a soul of one sex into a body of a different sex, by His Omniscience He would know the outcome, and God does not intentionally cause pain or suffering. He allows it by His Permissive Will, but He does not cause it. Since He is the only Creator of souls, He would have to intentionally create a soul of one

---

[42] Most Rev. Salvatore J. Cordileone and Most Rev. Michael C. Barber, S.J., *"The Body-Soul Unity of the Human Person"* (*September 29, 2023*), pg. 2.

[43] John Desilva Finley, "The Metaphysics of Gender: A Thomistic Approach," *The Thomist* 79 (2015): 585-614.

[44] St. Thomas Aquinas, *Summa Theologica*, I, q. 75, arts 1, 5, and 7, from https://www.newadvent.org/summa/1.htm.

sex and unite it to a body of the opposite sex. That too would be denying one of the defining characteristics of God, in this case, Omnibenevolence.

Another view proposed by Finley looks deeper into the philosophical notion of the "form" of physical entities.[45] Aristotle claimed that the soul is the 'form' of the body.[46] The Catholic Church affirmed this in 1312 AD, at the General Council of Vienne, when they wrote "...*we reject as erroneous to the Catholic faith any doctrine or opinion which rashly asserts that the substance of the rational and intellectual soul is not truly and of itself (per se) the form of the human body...*"[47]

In philosophy, the term 'form' means that characteristic of a thing which gives it a specific identity. It is the 'essence' of a thing. The 'form' is different from 'matter' of which substances are composed.[48] For example, bronze can be a lump in a foundry or, if made into a statue, its matter takes on a form and it becomes a statue. The statue is then a composite of form (which helps us recognize it as a statue) and matter of which the statue is composed.

---

[45] John Desilva Finley, ed., *Sexual Identity – The Harmony of Philosophy, Science, and Revelation.* (Steubenville, Ohio: Emmaus Road Publishing, 2022), 244-ff.

[46] S. Marc Cohen, Patricia Curd, and C.D.C Reeve, eds., *Readings in Ancient Greek Philosophy – From Thales to Aristotle*, 3rd ed. (Indianapolis: Hackett Publishing Company, 2005), 813.

[47] Jacques Dupuis, ed., *The Christian Faith in the Doctrinal Documents of the Catholic Church*, 7th Revised and Enlarged Edition, (New York: Alba House, 2001), 169-170.

[48] S. Marc Cohen, Patricia Curd, and C.D.C Reeve, *Readings in Ancient Greek Philosophy*, 944.

According to Aristotle, *"the soul first and foremost 'actualizes' matter: it gives it being, in the first place, and forms it to be a body of a certain kind – namely a living organism belonging to the species from which it came."*[49] Finley asserts that while a soul is not a body, it *"is something of a body"* and *"makes bodiliness exist and act as a certain kind of living unified thing."*[50] Further, he notes that, the soul is a spiritual principle, not material, and that the human being is a *"soul-body composite."* The soul *"actualizes"* the body and gives it structure that enables its proper human functions.[51]

Finally, as far as a philosophical approach, Finley asserts that the *"human soul is radically one with the body it animates. They come into being together as the embryonic human person, and naturally exist as one being throughout the person's life."*[52] He notes that the soul is spiritual, so it doesn't depend on matter for its existence, and its origin or source is God, our Creator. Taking all of the above into consideration leads one to conclude that sexuality *"is a matter of soul and body together,"* and *"it involves the body precisely because the soul is the **form** of the body." ."*[53] And, since the soul is the form of the body, each soul must, thus be consistent with the sex of the body it forms.

The soul actualizes the body, i.e., takes matter, and structures it into a living organism with certain capabilities. One of these is the ability to reproduce. *"Male and female are the two ways in which this*

---

[49] John Desilva Finley, *Sexual Identity,* 241.
[50] Ibid.
[51] John Desilva Finley, *Sexual Identity,* 242.
[52] John Desilva Finley, *Sexual Identity,* 244.
[53] John Desilva Finley, *Sexual Identity,* 245.

capacity is manifest in the human species."[54] "*It is the **person** that is sexed (soul **and** body), not the soul or matter in their own right.*" Pope Paul VI noted, "*Though made of body and soul, man is one.*"[55] Pope John Paul II considered sex to be a constitutive property of the body-soul unity.[56] Therefore, if souls are sexually differentiated, one could not put a female soul into a male body because by definition, the soul is the form of the body and is itself the cause of maleness or female-ness of the body.

One might argue that children are born with diseases and that must be willed by God, so how is "Gender Dysphoria" any different? The difference is, when a child is born with a disease, it is again by God's permissive will, which allows ontic evil such as disease, but does not cause it. These natural evils are rather the result of our fallen state of existence in which our originally perfect existence has been darkened by sin and all sorts of evils result. Then, one could say that God's permissive will allowed a person to be born with "Gender Dysphoria" if it is caused by a mental illness, but one could not say that God created a female soul in a male body.

Therefore, the claim that God put a female soul in a male body or vice-versa must be wrong.

Argument from Religion

Why only "male" and "female?" Why are there only two sexes? These questions lead us way back to the beginning in chapter one of

---

[54] John Desilva Finley, *Sexual Identity,* 246.

[55] Paul VI, *Gaudium et Spes,* n. 14.

[56] John Paul II, *Veritatis Splendor,* n. 48.

Genesis. There we are told that God created human beings *"in our image, after our likeness"* (Gen. 1:26) and *"God created mankind in his image, in the image of God he created them, male and female he created them"* (Gen. 1:27). We also learn that God said, *"be fertile and multiply"* (Gen. 1:28),[57] and that *"it is not good for the man to be alone."*[58]

What does all this mean with respect to "Gender Dysphoria." First, it shows God's intention to create **two sexes**. After all, why didn't God create only men, or only women, or some androgenous beings without any sexual constitutive properties? It has to do with man being created in the "image of God." God is Trinitarian in nature, <u>a communion</u> of three divine persons – Father, Son, and Holy Spirit. Being made in the image and likeness of God doesn't mean that man or woman "look like God" in a physical sense. Rather, we were created with intellect and will, and to be in communion with each other as God the Father, Son, and Holy Spirit are in the Trinity.

As Pope John Paul II, put it, *"To say that man is created in the image and likeness of God means that man is called to exist 'for' others, to become a gift."*[59] In addition, *"man and woman, created as a 'unity of the two' in their common humanity, are called to live in a communion of love, and in this way to mirror in the world the communion of love that is in God."*[60] Thus, it is only together that man and woman image the likeness of God. Apart, each is missing something, but together they find meaning outside of themselves.

---

[57] Catholic Biblical Association, *The Holy Bible,* Gen. 1:26,27,28.

[58] Catholic Biblical Association, *The Holy Bible,* Gen. 2:18.

[59] John Paul II, *Mulieris Dignitatem (August 15, 1988),* n. 7.

[60] Ibid.

Humans are, therefore, created to be in communion, in relationship with another, and to look outward, not to be focused on the self.

Second, it shows God's intent **IN** creating two sexes (reproduction). This is most evident in the way male and female bodies exhibit a complementarity. Specifically, the male body is designed to provide one of the two essential components required for human reproduction (the sperm). Similarly, the female body is designed to receive that component, to provide the other essential component (the ovum, or egg), and to provide the space and nutrient support for the developing human baby. Through this complementarity they complete each other. John Paul II notes, *"When both unite so intimately with each other that they become "one flesh…" this union carries within itself a particular awareness of the meaning of that body in the reciprocal self-gift of the persons."*[61] Note, there is no other component necessary for human reproduction.

So, another way that male and female image God is in their ability to create, or more specifically, to procreate. Acting together, in communion, a man and a woman, in a sincere gift of themselves can share in God's generative power and co-create another human being. When done in the context of a sacramental marriage, the child born of the one flesh union is another exemplar of the Trinitarian nature of God. As Augustine says,[62] *"if the love by which the Father loves the Son, and the Son loves the Father, ineffably demonstrates the communion of both, what is more suitable than that He should be*

---

[61] John Paul II, *Man and woman He created them*, 169.

[62] Augustine of Hippo, "On the Trinity," vol. 3, in *St. Augustin: On the Holy Trinity, Doctrinal Treatises, Moral Treatises*, P. Schaff (Ed.), & A. W. Haddan (Trans.), (Christian Literature Company, 1887), 219.

specially called love, who is the Spirit common to both?" Thus, as the love of the Father and Son, can be called the Holy Spirit, a child can be called the love of a man and a woman.

All of this is to say, that the process of attempting to change one's sex, causes such harm to the body that the person can no longer make an authentic gift of self to another human. As discussed in Part One, puberty blockers, hormone therapy, and sex "reassignment" surgery, can result in infertility. This results in an inability to love as God intended.

Morality and Gender Ideology

We live in a fallen world. Sin and corruption are the result of that real "primeval event"[63] in which man chose to follow his own will rather than follow God's Will. Although God desires only good for man, in choosing to disobey God, Adam lost the "original holiness"[64] with which he was created. It was in this fallen state that he and Eve bore children, who could not be born in holiness given the fallen state of their parents. Thus, the sin of Adam was and is propagated to all of his descendants, not as committed sin, but as contracted sin[65].

One might consider, looking at this event from a scientific point of view, that our first parents must have been created perfectly good. Their bodies, organs, senses, right down to their DNA,[66] must have

---

[63] CCC 390.
[64] CCC 375.
[65] CCC 404.
[66] Source unknown.

been perfect because "...*God saw everything that he had made, and behold, it was very good.*"[67] However, immediately after sin entered the world, man's body became subject to damage; thus, suffering and death entered the world. But, with each successive generation, man's DNA became progressively more damaged. Given the number of generations since that time, therefore, diseases and disorders are to be expected as falling within God's Permissive Will and as a result of that primeval act.

Psychiatrist Dr. Jack Drescher was one of the people on the American Psychiatric Association's Sexual and Gender Identity Disorders Working Group. This group sought to remove the gender variance, previously known as Gender Identity Disorder, from the Fifth Edition of the Diagnostic and Statistics Manual of Mental Disorders (DSM-5).[68] Their aim was to remove the concept of gender variance as a disorder. They would then replace it with the distress associated with "Gender Dysphoria" as the mental disorder. This begs the question as to who is to decide what is normal or moral? In Part One, we noted that mathematically speaking, "normal" means representative of the majority of the population and "ordered" means working according to the designed and intended function. Variation is not always good. This is where science cannot be the only voice.

In a 2010 publication, Drescher noted, somewhat ruefully, that "*Traditionally, religion has played a strong role in codifying socially*

---

[67] Catholic Biblical Association, *The Holy Bible*, Gen. 1:31).

[68] American Psychiatric Association, *Diagnostic and statistical manual of mental disorders* (5th ed.) (2013) https://doi.org/10.1176/appi.books. 9780890425596.

acceptable expressions of gender and sexuality."[69] And, in this author's view, that is rightfully so. But some in the fields of science and medicine have clear anti-religion biases as is obvious from his further statements, such as, "*An ill person was not necessarily responsible for his or her 'symptoms,' and, in the best of circumstances, would benefit from therapeutic compassion rather than religious judgment and condemnation*".[70] Nevertheless, it is not within human authority to define what is morally right or wrong. For each person there might be a different answer. That is where God comes in. Morality, of necessity, has been defined for man by God. In his discussion on morality in *Veritatis Splendor*, St. Pope John Paul II noted that although man has '*rightful autonomy,*' this "*…autonomy of reason cannot mean that reason itself creates values and moral norms.*" [71]

Only by following God's Commandments can we be sure the path we are on is correct. While we can come to know these through reason as they pertain to Natural Law, these have also been promulgated, as a great gift to mankind, and have come to us through the Sacred Scriptures.[72] This gift has been given in order to help man in his journey back to reconciliation with God, and to once again resemble the image of God. The Scriptures have been interpreted and explained by moral theologians and philosophers. Their content has remained unchanged over the several millennia since they were

---

[69] Drescher, Jack. "Queer Diagnoses: Parallels and Contrasts in the History of Homosexuality, Gender Variance, and the Diagnostic and Statistical Manual." *Archives of Sexual Behavior* 39.2 (2010): 427-60.

[70] Ibid.

[71] Pope John Paul II, *Veritatis Splendor* (August 6, 1993), n. 40.

[72] May, William E. (2003) An Introduction to Moral Theology. Second Ed. Indian: Our Sunday Visitor, Inc.

written, but their meaning is interpreted in every age. Again, St. Pope John Paul II wrote that: "*Man's genuine moral autonomy in no way means the rejection but rather the acceptance of the moral law, of God's command: "The Lord God gave this command to the man..." (Gen 2:16). Human freedom and God's law meet and are called to intersect, in the sense of man's free obedience to God and of God's completely gratuitous benevolence towards man.*"[73]

St. Pope John Paul II also discussed the contemporary argument that proposes a person's intentions are what determines whether an action is right or wrong, and that the consequences of an action make it right or wrong (i.e., the ends justifying the means). However, he dismisses these arguments as "*... not faithful to the Church's teaching, when they believe they can justify, as morally good, deliberate choices of kinds of behavior contrary to the commandments of the divine and natural law. These theories cannot claim to be grounded in the Catholic moral tradition.*"[74]

He notes that the "*...Catechism of the Catholic Church teaches, 'there are certain specific kinds of behavior that are always wrong to choose, because choosing them involves a disorder of the will, that is, a moral evil'. And Saint Thomas observes,*[75] "*it often happens that man acts with a good intention, but without spiritual gain, because he lacks a good will. Let us say that someone robs in order to feed the poor: in this case, even though the intention is good, the uprightness of the will is lacking. Consequently, no evil done with a good intention can be excused.*

---

[73] Pope John Paul II, *Veritatis Splendor*, n. 41.
[74] Ibid. n. 76.
[75] Ibid. n. 78.

According to St. Pope John Paul II, the morality of an act depends on the *"object"* chosen by the person's will, that is, <u>what</u> they choose to do. Some objects cannot be *"ordered to God"* because they are bad for the person. God's laws are all made to protect us from objects of our will that would harm us. *"Whatever is hostile to life itself, such as any kind of homicide, genocide, abortion... mutilation... all these and the like are a disgrace... and they are a negation of the honor due to the Creator."*[76]

The Church teaches of the existence of *"intrinsically evil"* acts through St. Paul who said *"Do not be deceived: neither the immoral, nor idolaters, nor adulterers, nor sexual perverts, nor thieves, nor the greedy, nor drunkards, nor revilers, nor robbers will inherit the Kingdom of God" (1 Cor 6:9-10).*[77] Further, *"If acts are intrinsically evil, a good intention or particular circumstances can diminish their evil, but they cannot remove it. They remain 'irremediably' evil acts; per se and in themselves they are not capable of being ordered to God and to the good of the person."*[78]

The Catholic Church states, *"The Christian vision of anthropology sees sexuality as a fundamental component of one's personhood. It is one of its mode [sic] of being, of manifesting itself, communicating with others, and of feeling, expressing and living human love."*[79] Therefore, *"Everyone, man and woman, should acknowledge and*

---

[76] Ibid. n. 80.

[77] Ibid. n.81.

[78] Ibid.

[79] Congregation for Catholic Education, *'Male and Female He Created Them' - Towards a Path of Dialogue on the Question of Gender Theory in Education* (February 2, 2019), n 4.

accept his sexual identity. Physical, moral, and spiritual difference and complementarity are oriented toward the goods of marriage and the flourishing of family life.[80]

Further, medical interventions such as puberty blockers, cross-sex hormones, and "SRS," "*are not morally justified either as attempts to repair a defect in the body or as attempts to sacrifice a part of the body for the sake of the whole.*"[81] These interventions "*do not respect the fundamental order of the human person as an intrinsic unity of body and soul, with a body that is sexually differentiated.*"[82]

Given the above from Sacred Scripture, the Catechism, and Papal and other Church Documents, it is justified to consider hormone therapy and "SRS" to be intrinsically evil because they are not ordered to the Will of God in that they refuse to accept what God has made. In addition, they reject the dignity of the human person and do harm to the person by introducing dangerous chemicals into the body, mutilating the body, and rendering human beings incapable of sexual reproduction and the fulfillment of God's command to be fruitful in marriage. Further, they do harm to the relationships within the families of those seeking to change their gender.

Special Considerations for Children

Before the age of reason, children cannot in any way be capable of understanding the ramifications of medical interventions for "Gender Dysphoria" for their future lives. Similarly, although

---

[80] CCC 2333.

[81] USCCB Committee on Doctrine, "*Doctrinal Note*," n.15.

[82] Ibid. n. 18.

adolescents are able to make rational choices, they cannot possibly comprehend what it means to lose the ability to bring their own children into the world.[83] Young human beings at the time of puberty are assaulted by hormones that make rational decisions much more difficult. This is why governments have age restrictions on driving, gun ownership, drinking, etc. Therefore, medical interventions for "Gender Dysphoria" in children and adolescents, i.e., especially before adulthood, are morally illicit.

As I noted in Part One, the vast majority of children with "Gender Dysphoria," desist by the time of puberty and adolescence. Thus, allowing early transitioning of children by hormones or other medical interventions may result in "*...transitioning someone who would not have otherwise persisted,*" which clearly violates the moral law.[84]

There are now instances where children suffering from "Gender Dysphoria" have been taken away from their parents because they have refused to affirm the child's desired gender. This too is against God's law. "*Reason tells us that two fundamental rights, which stem from the very nature of the family, must always be guaranteed and protected. Firstly, the family's right to be recognized as the primary pedagogical environment for the educational formation of children.*"[85] That is, the parents have the right and primary responsibility to educate their children and that carries with it ultimate authority over

---

[83] Tony N. Jelsma, "*An Attempt to Understand Gender and Gender Dysphoria: A Christian Approach,*" The American Scientific Affiliation (ASA) and the Canadian Scientific and Christian Association (CSC), November 2021, https://digitalcollections.dordt.edu/faculty_work.

[84] Ibid.

[85] Congregation for Catholic Education, "'Male and Female He Created Them,'" n. 37.

what they are taught and what they can do. Schools and educators outside the family by God's design are established in a subsidiary role to the nuclear family.

The Church also speaks to the aforementioned acts by governments to circumvent the rights of parents to decide matters for the welfare of their children – especially medical matters. Pius XII noted, "*What We say here must extend to the legal representative of one who is incapable of disposing of himself and his affairs: children before the age of reason…These legal representatives, established by a private decision or by public authority, have no other right over the body and life of their subordinates than themselves… They cannot therefore give the doctor permission to dispose of them outside these limits.*"[86]

Spiritual Warfare

As the Congregation for Catholic Education rightly noted, sexuality is at the core of our identity as human beings. The Congregation for the Doctrine of the Faith also observed, "*Sexuality characterizes man and woman not only on the physical level, but also on the psychological and spiritual, making its mark on each of their expressions. It… is a fundamental component of personality, one of its modes of being, of manifestation, of communicating with others, of feeling, of expressing and of living human love.*"[87]

---

[86] Pius XII, *Speech from Pope Pius XII,* Section II, Para 10.

[87] Congregation for the Doctrine of the Faith, "Letter on the Collaboration of Men and Woman in the Church and in the World" (2004), 4,

Given this, it would make a compelling target for attack if one wanted to confuse a person's perception of reality. One potential mechanism for "Gender Dysphoria" that would never be posited by secular sciences is the influence of the devil. A direct consequence of accepting the existence of God is the acknowledgment of a supernatural world that is hidden from our view. If one accepts the Sacred Scriptures, and likewise acknowledges that humans were created by God, it is equally plausible that God made other rational creatures, and we know them from the Scriptures as angels. The greatest gift of God to His rational creatures, humans included, is the freedom to choose what path they will take. With this free will, some of the angels, out of envy,[88] chose not to accept God's love. This began a time of spiritual warfare that continues to this day. If one accepts the Scriptures as true, then one must acknowledge the power of the devil and other demonic forces in the world. In fact, even Pope Francis acknowledged that *"gender ideology is demonic."*[89]

The goal of demons is to lead humans to sin and away from God, ultimately to eternal death. Their tactics are many and usually begin with lesser sins which lead to self-recrimination. Then, they tempt the individual to define themselves as a sinner, from which point other sins are easier to commit. One such entry point for "Gender Dysphoria" is likely to be pornography. Some men and women use

---

https://www.vatican.va/roman_curia/congregations/cfaith/documents/rc_con_cfaith_doc_20040731_collaboration_en.html.

[88] Wisdom of Solomon, 2:24.

[89] John-Henry Westen, "Austrian bishop: Pope Francis told me 'gender ideology is demonic," Life Site News, June 17, 2014, https://www.lifesitenews.com/news/austrianbishoppopefrancistoldmegenderideologyisdemonic.

pornography to derive sexual pleasure from images that allow them to achieve sexual orgasm. This reduces the persons viewed to objects of pleasure and takes from them their basic dignity as human beings. If a man or woman reduces sexuality to a selfish pleasure, it is not difficult to anticipate that a sexual addiction will follow, and that the addict could become enthralled with the idea of sexual pleasure obtained from viewing one's own body altered in form to represent the other gender. This would bring about a form of demonic possession in which the person is driven toward saying to God, I will choose my sex for my own pleasure to be different from what you assigned to me. This is a great sin and a direct attack by the devil on the human person on many levels.

Negative Effects of "Gender Dysphoria" on the Person and Family

In Part Two, the negative physical effects of hormone treatments were discussed. There are other, non-medical, effects that result from a person attempting to change their gender that are in the realm of sociology and especially of familial relationships. When a person decides to change their gender, they are not the only people affected by that choice. Others who love them, such as parents, siblings, and other family members and friends, are often thrown into confusion and suffering. The desire to love that person does not go away, but the person essentially does. Despite all reassurances that "I am still the same person," our gender is such a basic part of who we are and how we relate to others that nothing can ever be the same in the relationship when a person tries to change their gender by socially transitioning (wearing clothing of the opposite sex, changing one's name to one more representative of the opposite sex, etc.) or medically transitioning. Parents, siblings, and friends feel a profound sense of loss and sorrow.[90] I know this from speaking with the friends and family of the young man, my son's friend, whose desire to transition began my search for understanding that led to this book.

In addition, because "SRS" destroys healthy organs for sexual reproduction, the persons themselves lose the ability to have a natural family. This is always true for men, and sometimes true for women. Given evidence of cancers in the reproductive organs of women after "SRS," there are recommendations that the organs be removed during the surgery even though, being internal organs they do not have to be removed. If healthy organs of generation are removed, it brings into question the ability of the person to enter into a truly sacramental marriage since God commanded Adam and Eve to "Be fertile and multiply."[91]

The canon law section on Marriage states: *"Sterility neither prohibits nor nullifies marriage, without prejudice to the prescript of can. 1098."*[92] However, canon 1098 states *"A person contracts invalidly who enters into a marriage deceived by malice, perpetrated to obtain consent, concerning some quality of the other partner which by its very nature can gravely disturb the partnership of conjugal life."*[93] In other words, if someone has transitioned by surgery and is no longer

---

[90] Personal communication.

[91] Catholic Biblical Association, *The Holy Bible*, Gen. 1:28.

[92] Code of Canon Law, c. 1084, § 3 (Vatican website English Translation).

[93] Ibid., c. 1098.

capable of procreation, this must be made known to the person they intend to marry, or the marriage can be considered invalid. Thus, pursuing treatment for "Gender Dysphoria" is not something that is without collateral damage or direct damage to the individual. These social consequences also argue against pursuing gender changes.

Catholic Views Must Include Compassion

Although we have constructed a reasonable view of what emerges from the basic teachings of the Catechism, other Basic Truths are also vitally important to remember. First and foremost, *"Being in the image of God [every] human individual possesses the dignity of a person, who is not just something, but someone."* [94] We are called by our Creator to love, not just some, but all people.

In our current society, the outcomes for individuals with "Gender Dysphoria" are grim. Drescher notes that there is significant *"...suffering attendant to these patterns ..."*[95] Bartlett, et al. point out that *"[r]ejected by peers and often their own families, adolescents with GID may be caught in a downward spiral similar to that which is found among other adolescents who have suffered rejection..."*[96]

Also as noted by Drescher before DSM-V was promulgated, the *"...designation of gender identity disorders as mental disorders is not a license for stigmatization..."* One of Drescher's recommendations

---

[94] CCC 357.

[95] Drescher, Jack. "Queer Diagnoses," 427.

[96] Nancy H. Bartlett, Paul L. Vassey, and William M. Bukowski, "Is Gender Identity Disorder in Children a Mental Disorder?" *Sex Roles* 43.11-12 (2000): 753-85.

that should be embraced by all is: "*...opposing the stigma associated with psychiatric disorders and accessing mental health services...*"[97]

The Church too embraces these notions. In the Pastoral Letter by Archbishop Cordileone and Bishop Barber, they note, "*no one should suffer bullying, violence, insults, or unjust discrimination.*"[98] Further, "*Many faithful Catholics demonstrate solidarity with those suffering from gender dysphoria... and sincerely desire to respond in love to their sisters and brothers.*" However, as the bishops observe, compassion must also include relaying the truth in love to those affected. Not to acknowledge the truth is false compassion.

What Can the Church Do to Help Our Brothers and Sisters Who Experience This Affliction?

God loves every human being individually. Those with mental disorders, physical diseases, and those who have none of those issues. He desires our flourishing, which is not typically the case for those with "Gender Dysphoria," especially those who go on to medical interventions as discussed in Parts One and Two of this book. We have to be especially careful not to judge those who are suffering from "Gender Dysphoria."[99] This is not something one chooses. Rather, we should seek to "*...accompany them by acknowledging their*

---

[97] Jack Drescher, "Queer Diagnoses," 427.

[98] Most Rev. Salvatore J. Cordileone and Most Rev. Michael C. Barber, S.J., "*The Body-Soul Unity*, pg. 2.

[99] The Most Rev. Allen H. Vigneron, "*The Good News About God's Plan*," pg. 6.

pain, listening to them, making sure they know they are heard, and assuring them of God's personal love for them."[100]

Just as there are genetic predispositions to addiction, that with recognition, love, and care can be managed, some mental illnesses, such as depression, are addressable with psychological or pharmacological interventions. Science should seek to cure "Gender Dysphoria" by generating better knowledge of its causes and encouraging research into psychological and/or pharmacological methods of treatment that aim to bring the mind into conformance with the body, or at least reduce the discomfort and stress associated with "Gender Dysphoria."

The suffering of individuals with "Gender Dysphoria" leads this author to call on the Church to support ethical studies of "Gender Dysphoria" towards understanding the issues and alleviating the suffering of the people who endure it. It also leads to a call for pastoral care of such individuals who, like the lepers in the time of Christ, are often cast out from society to live on their own.

Conclusions to Part Three

We live in a fallen world. Illness, natural disasters, and moral evil are all part of it. To deny those facts is to deny reality itself. Given the facts as discussed above, **we are led to conclude that gender "reassignment" is contrary to the laws of God as we understand them**, from Church teaching as revealed in the Bible, from the Church Fathers and Doctors, from the Magisterium as represented by the Pope, and from the Catechism. While that is the truth, it does

---

[100] Ibid., pg. 7.

not address the objective reality that there are those who feel that, by no choice of their own, they have "Gender Dysphoria." However, they do have a choice as to whether to act upon those feelings. Celibacy, chastity, and joining our suffering with that of Christ as an offering for others are some of the goods that our Faith teach in such circumstances.

Like someone born without a limb, or with a chronic disease such as Cystic Fibrosis, Clinical Depression, or Cerebral Palsy, to name just a few, a person with feelings of "Gender Dysphoria" should be treated with compassion and helped to live a life in which they do not act on those feelings, as difficult as that may be.

The Committee on Doctrine of the United States Conference of Catholic Bishops, in their *Doctrinal Note on the Moral Limits to Technological Manipulation of the Human Body*, observe that modern medical technologies have many positive uses, but also pose the danger of harming the patients they are intended to help.[101] They note that, *"Careful moral discernment is needed to determine which possibilities should be realized and which should not, in order to promote the good of the human person."*

What is morally right is not the purview of science or medicine. It is the purview of philosophy, ethics, and ultimately religion. What human can say with authority, "This is right and that is wrong?" Man will always have an ulterior motive. The Judeo-Christian values upon which the laws of many civilized nations were founded, are not the creation of men. They reflect the goodness of Creation and the dignity of the human person as willed by God. They espouse *"the*

---

[101] USCCB Committee on Doctrine, *"Doctrinal Note,"* n.1.

basic condition for love of neighbor; and at the same time they are proof of that love."[102] Humankind left to itself will always serve itself. Allowing each person to choose what he or she autonomously believes to be right is anarchy. No civilization so inclined will remain civil for long.

Morality, as defined by God in the goodness of Creation and human dignity, enables human beings to fulfill ourselves and our destiny, which is true happiness in Him.

Proposed Actions from Part Three:

-   At the level of the Vatican and Catholic Universities, the Church should:

    o   support studies seeking to understand the etiology of "Gender Dysphoria"
    o   support studies to find moral and effective treatments that respect the human person and restore the person to mental health

-   At the level of Dioceses and Parishes:

    o   seek ways to shelter, minister to, and pastor individuals with "Gender Dysphoria" like it does the poor and indigent.

---

[102] John Paul II, *Veritatis Splendor* (August 6, 1993), n. 13.

ENDNOTE

I end with quotes from two of the Popes who have had the greatest impact on our understanding of human anthropology in the modern Church.

St. Pope Paul VI noted, "man cannot find true happiness towards which he aspires with all his being other than in respect of the laws written by God in his very nature, laws which he must observe with intelligence and love."[1]

St. Pope John Paul II wrote, "Faith and reason are like two wings on which the human spirit rises to the contemplation of truth; and God has placed in the human heart a desire to know the truth-in a word, to know himself-so that, by knowing and loving God, men and women may also come to the fullness of truth about themselves."[2]

---

[1] St. Paul VI, *Humanae Vitae* (July 25, 1968), n.31.
[2] John Paul II, *Fides et Ratio* (September 14, 1998), Intro.

INDEX

www.ingramcontent.com/pod-product-compliance
Lightning Source LLC
Chambersburg PA
CBHW070040100426
42740CB00013B/2740